T0292265

The Pocket Guide to Medical Retina

Ophthalmology Pocket Guides
Series

SERIES EDITOR, RICHARD L. LINDSTROM

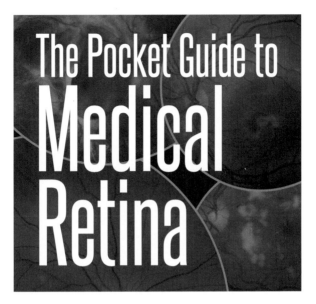

The Pocket Guide to Medical Retina

EDITORS

Jason Hsu, MD
Co-Director of Retina Research
Retina Service of Wills Eye Hospital
Associate Professor of Clinical Ophthalmology
Sidney Kimmel Medical College
Thomas Jefferson University
Philadelphia, Pennsylvania

Allen Chiang, MD
Retina Service of Wills Eye Hospital
Associate Professor of Clinical Ophthalmology
Sidney Kimmel Medical College
Thomas Jefferson University
Philadelphia, Pennsylvania

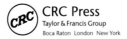

CRC Press
Taylor & Francis Group
Boca Raton London New York

CRC Press is an imprint of the
Taylor & Francis Group, an **informa** business

First published 2021 by SLACK Incorporated

Published 2024 by CRC Press
2385 NW Executive Center Drive, Suite 320, Boca Raton FL 33431

and by CRC Press
4 Park Square, Milton Park, Abingdon, Oxon, OX14 4RN

CRC Press is an imprint of Taylor & Francis Group, LLC

© 2021 Taylor & Francis Group, LLC

Cover Artist: Katherine Christie

Library of Congress Cataloging-in-Publication Data

Names: Hsu, Jason, editor. | Chiang, Allen, editor.
Title: The pocket guide to medical retina / [edited by] Jason Hsu, Allen Chiang.
Description: Thorofare, NJ : SLACK Incoporated, 2020. | Includes bibliographical references and index.
Identifiers: LCCN 2020017636 (print) | ISBN 9781630916329 (paperback)
Subjects: MESH: Retinal Diseases--therapy | Retinal Diseases--diagnosis Handbook
Classification: LCC RE551 (print) | LCC RE551 (ebook) | NLM WW 39 | DDC 617.7/35--dc23
LC record available at https://lccn.loc.gov/2020017636

ISBN: 9781630916329 (pbk)
ISBN: 9781003525790 (ebk)

DOI: 10.1201/9781003525790

DEDICATION

To my colleagues at Wills Eye and Mid Atlantic Retina
whose dedication to teaching, patient care, and
research motivates me on a daily basis. It is a privilege to
work with so many esteemed leaders and future leaders
of our field.

To my current and past trainees, many of whom have
contributed to this book, for their camaraderie through the
years. Much of what I have accomplished would not have been
possible without your dedication to our
many research endeavors.

Above all, to my family, for their constant love and support. First
and foremost, to my wife, Vatinee, for always being my
shoulder to lean on. To my children, Aidan, Ethan, and Bryan,
for all the joy they have brought into this world. And to my
parents, Edward and Phyllis, for the values
they instilled in me.

—*Jason Hsu, MD*

To my past teachers and mentors, for their dedication, guidance,
and professional support.

To my colleagues at Wills Eye Physicians—Mid Atlantic Retina
and Wills Eye Hospital, with whom it has been a privilege and
honor to partner with in caring for patients, advancing
retina research, and training future leaders in
ophthalmology and retina.

To the fellows and residents at Wills who continually inspire
me to be a better teacher and physician, and to all my patients
who have trusted me with the honor of fighting
for their sight.

To my parents, Richard and Catherine, for raising and caring for me with an unconditional love, and leading exemplary lives for their children to follow.

Most of all to my wife, Helen, who has always supported me with inexplicable love and grace, and to my children, Emmeline, Jonathan, and Andrew, who have made our lives immeasurably richer and more joyful.

—*Allen Chiang, MD*

Contents

ACKNOWLEDGMENTS

We are extraordinarily grateful for the contributions of so many of our colleagues. Without them, this book would not have been possible. Many of the senior authors are our partners, esteemed colleagues at Wills Eye and multiple academic institutions, and former fellows and residents. It has been a great privilege to work with so many talented and eminent clinicians. However, much of the "grunt" work was accomplished by the chapter co-authors who were often retina fellows, residents, and medical students. We are deeply indebted to them for taking up the challenge and setting such a high bar. Without a doubt, the high-quality images in this book would not have been possible without the many outstanding staff and ophthalmic photographers at our various institutions. We wish to thank them for their services as well.

This book would never have been created without the insight of Tony Schiavo, editing guidance of Joseph Lowery, and the dedication of the whole team at SLACK Incorporated's Health Care Books and Journals division. We are sincerely grateful for their efforts in creating such an amazing finished product.

Above all, we wish to acknowledge our families who have put up with our late-night editing and obsessive-compulsive behavior in trying to perfect this pocket guide.

ABOUT THE EDITORS

Jason Hsu, MD is Co-Director of Retina Research at the Retina Service of Wills Eye Hospital and Associate Professor of Ophthalmology at the Sidney Kimmel Medical College of Thomas Jefferson University. He received his medical degree from the University of Pennsylvania School of Medicine and was elected to the Alpha Omega Alpha Medical Honor Society, followed by an ophthalmology residency at the University of Pennsylvania, Scheie Eye Institute, and a vitreoretinal surgery fellowship at Wills Eye Hospital. He is currently also a partner at Wills Eye Physicians—Mid Atlantic Retina.

Dr. Hsu is an active member of the Retina Society, American Society of Retina Specialists (ASRS), American Academy of Ophthalmology (AAO), and Association for Research in Vision and Ophthalmology (ARVO). He serves as Chair of the Retina Society's Website and Communications Committee and is a Retina/Vitreous committee member of the AAO Ophthalmic News and Education (ONE) Network. He has received the ASRS Honor Award, ASRS Senior Honor Award, and the AAO Achievement Award.

His academic accomplishments include over 200 peer-reviewed publications, editorials, book chapters, and scientific abstracts. Dr. Hsu has presented scientific papers at dozens of national and international ophthalmic conferences in addition to serving as a course instructor and symposium chair at the annual AAO meeting. He is a member of the editorial board for *Retinal Cases and Brief Reports*, *Retina Today*, and *Retina Specialist*. He serves as section editor for *Current Opinion in Ophthalmology* as well as ASRS's *Retina Times* and is a peer reviewer for all the major ophthalmology journals. In addition, Dr. Hsu has been principal investigator or co-investigator at Wills Eye Hospital for many national and international clinical trials pertaining to age-related macular degeneration, diabetic retinopathy, uveitis, and retinal vein occlusions.

Allen Chiang, MD is Associate Professor of Ophthalmology at the Sidney Kimmel Medical College of Thomas Jefferson University and is an active member of the Retina Service of Wills Eye Hospital. He received his medical degree from New York University with Alpha Omega Alpha honors, followed by a residency in ophthalmology at the Stein Eye Institute at University of California, Los Angeles, where he earned the Resident Awards for excellence in surgery and clinical research. He then completed a fellowship in retinal diseases and surgery at Wills Eye Hospital and was the recipient of the William Tasman, MD Fellow award. After practicing in the San Francisco Bay Area, he returned to Philadelphia and is currently a partner at Wills Eye Physicians— Mid Atlantic Retina.

His academic accomplishments include over 80 peer-reviewed journal articles, editorials, textbook chapters, and scientific abstracts. Dr. Chiang serves on the Peer Review Committee of Wills Eye Hospital, several committees of Wills Eye Physicians— Mid Atlantic Retina, the retina/vitreous section of the editorial board for the AAO ONE Network, and as an ad-hoc reviewer for multiple ophthalmology journals. He is actively engaged in clinical research and is the principal investigator on multiple clinical trials for conditions such as macular degeneration and diabetic retinopathy. He is a member of the Retina Society, ASRS, AAO, ARVO, and Vit Buckle Society, and is a past ASRS Honor Award recipient.

CONTRIBUTING AUTHORS

Musa Abdelaziz, MD (Chapter 7)
The Retina Group of Washington
Washington, DC

Christopher M. Aderman, MD (Chapters 3 and 8)
EyeHealth Northwest
Portland, Oregon

Roozbeh Akhtari, MD (Chapter 9)
Glaucoma Fellowship
Emory University
Atlanta, Georgia

Tomas S. Aleman, MD (Chapters 5 and 6)
Scheie Eye Institute
Perelman Center for Advanced Medicine
Department of Ophthalmology
University of Pennsylvania
Philadelphia, Pennsylvania

Ferhina S. Ali, MD, MPH (Chapters 2 and 6)
Sierra Eye Associates
Reno, Nevada

Paul S. Baker, MD (Chapters 4 and 9)
Pennsylvania Retina Specialists
Camp Hill, Pennsylvania

Alok S. Bansal, MD (Chapters 1 and 4)
Clinical Assistant Professor of Ophthalmology
The University of California, San Francisco
San Francisco, California

Cagri G. Besirli, MD, PhD (Chapter 6)
Department of Ophthalmology and Visual Sciences
University of Michigan
Ann Arbor, Michigan

Durga S. Borkar, MD (Chapter 2)
Assistant Professor of Ophthalmology
Vitreoretinal Surgery and Diseases
Duke University Eye Center
Durham, North Carolina

Kevin Broderick, MD (Chapter 7)
The Retina Group of Washington
Chevy Chase, Maryland

Jordan D. Deaner, MD (Chapters 1 and 2)
Wills Eye Hospital
Philadelphia, Pennsylvania
Cole Eye Institute
Cleveland Clinic
Cleveland, Ohio

Michael Dollin, MD, FRCSC (Chapters 1 and 6)
The Ottawa Hospital
University of Ottawa Eye Institute
Ottawa, Ontario, Canada

James P. Dunn, MD (Chapters 3 and 4)
Director, Uveitis Unit
Retina Division
Wills Eye Hospital
Professor of Ophthalmology
Sidney Kimmel Medical College
Thomas Jefferson University
Philadelphia, Pennsylvania

Sunir J. Garg, MD, FACS (Chapter 3)
Professor of Ophthalmology
Co-Director Retina Research Unit
Retina Service of Wills Eye Hospital
Thomas Jefferson University
Philadelphia, Pennsylvania
Editor in Chief
Retina Times
Chicago, Illinois

Sean T. Garrity, MD (Chapters 4 and 9)
New England Eye Center
Boston, Massachusetts

Adam T. Gerstenblith, MD (Chapters 4 and 8)
Mid Atlantic Retina Specialists
Hagerstown, Maryland

Kalla A. Gervasio, MD (Chapter 3)
Department of Ophthalmology
Wills Eye Hospital
Philadelphia, Pennsylvania

Shilpa Gulati, MD, MS (Chapter 2)
New England Eye Center
Ophthalmic Consultants of Boston
Boston, Massachusetts

Allen C. Ho, MD, FACS (Chapters 1 and 6)
Attending Surgeon and Director of Retina Research
Wills Eye Hospital
Professor of Ophthalmology
Thomas Jefferson University
Mid Atlantic Retina
Philadelphia, Pennsylvania

Samuel K. Steven Houston III, MD (Chapters 2 and 9)
Florida Retina Institute
Lake Mary, Florida

Sasha Hubschman, MD (Chapters 2 and 3)
Department of Ophthalmology
Bascom Palmer Eye Institute
Miller School of Medicine
University of Miami
Miami, Florida

Thomas Jenkins, MD (Chapter 2)
Retina Institute of Virginia
Richmond, Virginia

Sundeep K. Kasi, MD (Chapters 1 and 4)
The Retina Group of Washington
Washington, DC

Ashley Khalili, MD (Chapter 2)
Northwell Health
Great Neck, New York

M. Ali Khan, MD (Chapters 1 and 7)
Retina Service of Wills Eye Hospital
Assistant Professor of Ophthalmology
Sidney Kimmel Medical College
Thomas Jefferson University
Philadelphia, Pennsylvania

Michael A. Klufas, MD (Chapters 6 and 7)
Retina Service of Wills Eye Hospital
Assistant Professor of Ophthalmology
Thomas Jefferson University
Philadelphia, Pennsylvania

Raymond Ko, MD, FRCSC, BSc (Chapter 6)
The Ottawa Hospital
University of Ottawa Eye Institute
Ottawa, Ontario, Canada

Hannah Levin, BS (Chapters 7 and 8)
Wills Eye Hospital
Thomas Jefferson University
Philadelphia, Pennsylvania

Nikolas J. S. London, MD (Chapter 3)
Retina Consultants
San Diego, California

Douglas R. Matsunaga, MD (Chapters 3 and 6)
Wills Eye Hospital
Philadelphia, Pennsylvania

Sonia Mehta, MD (Chapters 3 and 4)
Wills Eye Hospital
Philadelphia, Pennsylvania

Phoebe L. Mellen, MD (Chapters 2 and 6)
Wills Eye Hospital
Philadelphia, Pennsylvania

Eugene A. Milder, MD (Chapter 1)
North Carolina Retina Associates
Raleigh, North Carolina

Anthony Obeid, MD (Chapter 7)
Wills Eye Hospital
Philadelphia, Pennsylvania

Carl H. Park, MD (Chapters 2 and 6)
Retina Service of Wills Eye Hospital
Assistant Professor
Thomas Jefferson University
Philadelphia, Pennsylvania

Samir Patel, MD (Chapter 6)
Wills Eye Hospital
Mid Atlantic Retina
Thomas Jefferson University
Philadelphia, Pennsylvania

Travis J. Peck, MD (Chapter 2)
Wills Eye Hospital
Philadelphia, Pennsylvania

John D. Pitcher III, MD (Chapters 1 and 9)
Vice President
Eye Associates of New Mexico
Medical Director
Vision Research Center
Assistant Professor of Ophthalmology
University of New Mexico
Albuquerque, New Mexico

Ehsan Rahimy, MD (Chapters 1 and 7)
Palo Alto Medical Foundation
Palo Alto, California

David C. Reed, MD (Chapter 2)
Ophthalmic Consultants of Boston
Boston, Massachusetts

Carl D. Regillo, MD (Chapters 2 and 7)
Director
Retina Service of Wills Eye Hospital
Professor of Ophthalmology
Thomas Jefferson University
Philadelphia, Pennsylvania

David Y. Rhee, MD (Chapters 2 and 9)
Partner
Long Island Vitreoretinal Consultants
Clinical Assistant Professor of Ophthalmology
Hofstra University
Retina Department
Northwell Health Hospital System
Long Island, New York

Chirag P. Shah, MD, MPH (Chapters 1 and 9)
Ophthalmic Consultants of Boston
Assistant Professor
Tufts University School of Medicine
Lecturer
Harvard Medical School
Boston, Massachusetts

Carol L. Shields, MD (Chapter 10)
Director
Ocular Oncology Service
Wills Eye Hospital
Philadelphia, Pennsylvania

Meera D. Sivalingam, MD (Chapter 3)
Ophthalmology Resident
Wills Eye Hospital
Thomas Jefferson University
Philadelphia, Pennsylvania

Elizabeth Maureen Sledz, MD (Chapter 9)
University of New Mexico
School of Medicine
Class of 2020, MD Candidate
Albuquerque, New Mexico

Rebecca R. Soares, MD, MPH (Chapter 4)
Ophthalmology Resident
Wills Eye Residency Program at Jefferson
Philadelphia, Pennsylvania

Mohamed K. Soliman, MD, MSc (Chapter 1)
Department of Ophthalmology
Assiut University Hospitals
Faculty of Medicine
Assiut University
Assiut, Egypt

Jayanth Sridhar, MD (Chapters 2 and 3)
Assistant Professor of Clinical Ophthalmology
University of Miami
Miami, Florida

Maxwell S. Stem, MD (Chapter 3)
Pennsylvania Retina Specialists
State College, Pennsylvania

Philip P. Storey, MD, MPH (Chapter 3)
Austin Retina
Austin, Texas

Daniel Su, MD (Chapter 3)
Retina-Vitreous Associates Medical Group
Los Angeles, California

Katherine E. Talcott, MD (Chapters 2 and 3)
Cole Eye Institute
Cleveland Clinic
Cleveland, Ohio

Matthew Trese, DO, MA (Chapters 4 and 6)
Beaumont Eye Institute
William Beaumont School of Medicine
Oakland University
Royal Oak, Michigan

Joshua H. Uhr, MD (Chapter 3)
Wills Eye Hospital
Thomas Jefferson University
Philadelphia, Pennsylvania

Priya Sharma Vakharia, MD (Chapters 1 and 9)
The Retina Group of Washington
Greenbelt, Maryland

James F. Vander, MD (Chapters 6 and 8)
Attending Surgeon
Retina Service of Wills Eye Hospital
Clinical Professor of Ophthalmology
Thomas Jefferson University
Philadelphia, Pennsylvania

Michael J. Venincasa, MD (Chapter 2)
Bascom Palmer Eye Institute
Miami, Florida

Eric D. Weichel, MD (Chapter 7)
Georgetown University
Washington Hospital Center
Washington, DC

Turner D. Wibbelsman, BS (Chapters 6 and 7)
Retina Service of Wills Eye Hospital
Philadelphia, Pennsylvania

Andre J. Witkin, MD (Chapters 4 and 9)
New England Eye Center
Boston, Massachusetts

Connie M. Wu, MD (Chapters 4 and 7)
Wills Eye Hospital
Philadelphia, Pennsylvania

Thomas J. Wubben, MD, PhD (Chapter 4)
Department of Ophthalmology and Visual Sciences
Kellogg Eye Center
University of Michigan
Ann Arbor, Michigan

David Xu, MD (Chapters 4 and 8)
Retina Service of Wills Eye Hospital
Thomas Jefferson University
Philadelphia, Pennsylvania

Prashant Yadav, MD, FRCS, FACS (Chapter 10)
Staff Ophthalmologist
Ocular Oncology Service
Wills Eye Hospital
Philadelphia, Pennsylvania

INTRODUCTION

This book is designed to provide individuals who are in training as well as comprehensive ophthalmologists and optometrists who are in practice with an easily navigable guide to a broad spectrum of vitreoretinal diseases. It is intended to be a concise yet thorough text that is systematically organized to provide a quick reference and high-yield learning. In addition, the book is image heavy to aid in pattern recognition and recall of relevant clinical information. Many of the images include markings to indicate salient features and teach readers how to interpret various diagnostics.

1

Macular Diseases

NON-EXUDATIVE (DRY) AGE-RELATED MACULAR DEGENERATION

Jordan D. Deaner, MD and
Allen C. Ho, MD, FACS

- Constitutes 85% to 90% of age-related macular degeneration (AMD). Drusen are the hallmark lesions, however retinal pigment epithelial (RPE) hyperpigmentation and atrophy may also be present.
- Oxidative stress is the suspected disease mechanism, resulting in photoreceptor toxicity, lipofuscin accumulation in RPE, drusen formation, and choriocapillaris atrophy.

Hsu J, Chiang A, eds. *The Pocket Guide to Medical Retina* (pp 1-38).
© 2021 Taylor & Francis Group.

Risk Factors

- Modifiable risk factors: smoking tobacco, hypertension, diet, physical activity, cardiovascular disease, hypercholesterolemia, obesity, and UV protection
- Non-modifiable risk factors: age (risk increases >3-fold in those >75 years old), genetic susceptibility (eg, complement factor H, *ARMS2*), female gender, Caucasian race, hyperopia, family history, light color irides

Signs and Symptoms

Decreased vision, metamorphopsia, micropsia, central scotoma

Exam Findings

- Drusen size: small (<63 μm), intermediate (63 to 124 μm), large (>124 μm)—for reference, retinal veins at optic disc margin are approximately 125 μm in diameter
- Drusenoid pigment epithelial detachments (PED) may arise from coalesced drusen (>350 μm)
- RPE granularity or stippling—RPE (geographic) atrophy (Figure 1-1A)

Staging of AMD as Defined by the Age-Related Eye Disease Study

- Early AMD: many small drusen or few (<10) intermediate drusen; risk of progression to advanced AMD is 1.3% over the 5-year period in the Age-Related Eye Disease Study (AREDS)
- Intermediate AMD: 10 or more intermediate drusen, a single large druse; risk of progression to advanced AMD is 18%
- Advanced AMD: presence of either geographic atrophy (GA) or choroidal neovascularization (CNV)

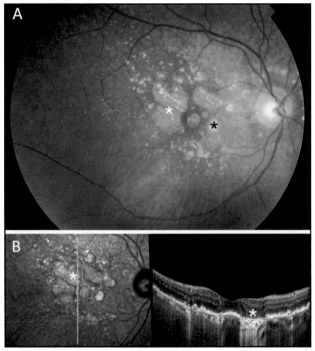

Figure 1-1. Dry AMD. (A) Color fundus photograph demonstrating areas of well-defined GA (white *) associated with many medium and large (black *) drusen. The choroidal vessels are well visualized in the areas of atrophy. (B) Infrared fundus image and OCT show areas of well demarcated GA (*).

Testing

- Optical coherence tomography (OCT): focal sub-RPE deposits correlate to drusen; loss of RPE and associated outer retinal structures correlate to GA (Figure 1-1B)
- OCT angiography (OCT-A): This dye-less imaging modality can identify CNV in a noninvasive manner.

- Fluorescein angiography (FA): Drusen typically show early blocking and late staining, but no leakage; GA presents as a transmission window defect without leakage; CNV will show leakage.
- Fundus autofluorescence (FAF): Drusen are classically hyperautofluorescent due to over-accumulation of lipofuscin within RPE cells, while GA appears as marked hypo-autofluorescence. Increased autofluorescence at borders of GA is associated with increased rate of progression.

Differential Diagnosis

Adult-onset foveomacular vitelliform dystrophy, Best disease, pattern dystrophy, central serous retinopathy, drug induced maculopathy (chloroquine, hydroxychloroquine)

Management

- Patients need to be educated on symptoms of CNV development including acute metamorphopsia, decreased vision, paracentral, or central scotoma.
  - Eyes with large soft drusen or RPE hyperpigmentation are at higher risk for development of CNV.
  - Home monitoring for CNV with either Amsler grid or a digital system such as ForeSeeHome which is approved by the Food and Drug Administration (FDA)
- Address modifiable risk factors such as healthy diet (leafy dark green vegetables and omega-3 fatty acids) and smoking cessation (most important modifiable risk factor)
- Low vision consultation for severe visual impairment
- Dietary supplementation
  - Original AREDS formula, recommended for patients with intermediate AMD or worse,[1] showed a 25% risk reduction in progression to advanced AMD over a 5-year period and 19% risk reduction of moderate vision loss.

This benefit continued at 10 years with 44% placebo vs 34% supplement patients with advanced AMD (27% risk reduction).

- ○ AREDS II study[2] showed the addition of lutein and zeaxanthin, docosahexaenoic acid (DHA) and eicosapentaenoic acid (EPA), or both, did not yield any additional risk reduction. However, lutein and zeaxanthin replaced beta carotene due to an increased risk of lung cancer in former smokers who took beta carotene.
- ○ AREDS II formula: 500 mg vitamin C, 400 IU vitamin E, 10 mg lutein, 2 mg zeaxanthin, 80 mg zinc, 2 mg copper

Wet Age-Related Macular Degeneration

Priya Sharma Vakharia, MD and
Chirag P. Shah, MD, MPH

- CNV typically develops in eyes with pre-existing dry AMD, which can lead to permanent visual impairment if not treated.
- Associated with older age, family history, genetics, and smoking; may also be associated with obesity and cardiovascular disease

Signs and Symptoms

Metamorphopsia, decreased vision, or scotoma

Exam Findings

Subretinal and/or intraretinal fluid, subretinal and/or intraretinal hemorrhage, gray membrane, lipid exudates, fibrovascular pigment epithelial detachment, associated with pre-existing drusen, atrophy, and retinal pigment epithelium changes (Figures 1-2A, 1-3A, and 1-3C)

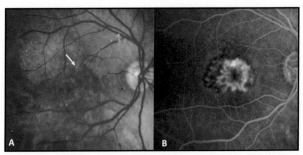

Figure 1-2. (A) Fundus photo demonstrating intraretinal and subretinal hemorrhage (arrow), associated with wet AMD. (B) FA with a well-defined hyperfluorescent lesion typical of classic CNV.

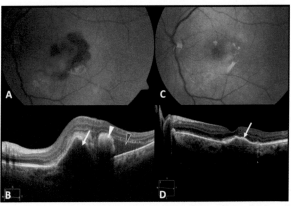

Figure 1-3. (A) Fundus photo demonstrating hemorrhage, fluid, and exudate, characteristic of wet AMD. (B) Corresponding OCT shows subretinal hemorrhage (white arrowhead), subretinal fluid (red arrowhead), and RPE detachment (white arrow). After 1 year of monthly anti-VEGF treatments, fundus photo (C) demonstrates resolution of hemorrhage and OCT (D) shows resolution of subretinal fluid and hemorrhage as well as a more compact retinal pigment epithelium detachment (white arrow).

Testing

- OCT: reveals presence of a CNV complex with intraretinal or subretinal fluid (Figures 1-3B and 1-3D)
- FA: Shows early hyperfluorescence and late leakage in the area of the CNV (Figure 1-2B). This can be associated with a classic or occult appearance.
- Indocyanine green angiography: Ancillary test to visualize the CNV complex, particularly helpful for occult CNV, polypoidal lesions, or when hemorrhage is present. Visualization is enhanced because indocyanine green is highly protein-bound and a longer wavelength is used.
- OCT angiography: noninvasive method of angiography which can reveal the CNV

Differential Diagnosis

Central serous chorioretinopathy, polypoidal choroidal vasculopathy, myopic CNV, idiopathic CNV, pattern dystrophy, vitelliform dystrophy, ocular histoplasmosis syndrome, angioid streaks and associated CNV, macular telangiectasia, chorioretinitis

Management

- Intravitreal anti-vascular endothelial growth factor (VEGF) injections decrease drive for abnormal blood vessel growth and reduce leakage from CNV.
  - Current standard of care with several different anti-VEGF medications currently available
    - Ranibizumab: Recombinant humanized monoclonal antibody fragment to VEGF. FDA-approved for treatment of wet AMD, based on results of pivotal ANCHOR and MARINA trials.[5,6]
    - Bevacizumab: Full-length humanized anti-VEGF antibody that is used off-label to treat macular degeneration. Was shown to be noninferior to

ranibizumab in the Comparison of AMD Treatment Trials (CATT).[7]

- Aflibercept: Fusion protein consisting of VEGF receptors 1 and 2 fused to Fc portion of IgG. FDA-approved for treatment of wet AMD; noninferior to ranibizumab in pivotal VIEW1 and VIEW2 trials.[4]
- Brolucizumab: Humanized single-chain antibody fragment that binds all isoforms of VEGF-A. FDA-approved for treatment of wet AMD: noninferior to aflibercept in pivotal HARRIER and HAWK trials.[3]
- Pegaptanib: Modified oligonucleotide which binds with and inactivates extracellular VEGF. First anti-VEGF therapy to be FDA-approved for wet AMD, demonstrating efficacy in the VISION trial.[8] Rarely used due to development of more effective drugs.
  ○ Treatment paradigms for injections
    - Monthly or fixed-interval dosing (based on landmark clinical trials)
    - Pro re nata (PRN): As needed when clinical or diagnostic evidence of activity, such as hemorrhage, macular edema on OCT or decreased vision. This method requires strict monthly monitoring to ensure no disease activity.
    - Treat-and-extend: injection at each visit but gradual lengthening of treatment intervals until signs of exudation are noted; interval is then shortened.
- Laser photocoagulation: causes local destruction of CNV
  ○ Limited efficacy and can have significant visual sequalae since retina overlying CNV is also damaged; rarely used in anti-VEGF era except occasionally for extrafoveal CNV
- Photodynamic therapy (PDT): FDA-approved treatment that involves injecting a photosensitive chemical (verteporfin) and activating it over CNV using a 689 nm laser in an

attempt to selectively induce CNV regression without damaging overlying retina

- ◦ Demonstrated to slow progression compared to natural history, but inferior to anti-VEGF therapy and is now rarely employed as monotherapy but may be used in combination with anti-VEGF for treatment resistant cases and is particularly helpful in polypoidal choroidal vasculopathy
- Pars plana vitrectomy (PPV)
  - ◦ With subretinal TPA: may be used in patients with thick submacular hemorrhage involving the fovea to liquefy and displace the hemorrhage
  - ◦ With extraction of CNV: largely historical and rarely used due to overall lack of efficacy and advent of anti-VEGF treatment

EPIRETINAL MEMBRANE (MACULAR PUCKER)

Sundeep K. Kasi, MD

- Growth of fibrocellular tissue on surface of retina causing disruption and wrinkling of macular contour
- Most frequently age-related and due in part to vitreous detachment, but must look for retinal tears, prior ocular surgery, and history of vein occlusion, inflammation or trauma
- Affects 2% of patients >50 years old and 20% of patients >75 years old. Ten to twenty percent bilateral but often asymmetric.

Signs and Symptoms

Decreased vision, distortion, metamorphopsia, and/or macropsia

Exam Findings

Reflective sheen over macula with effacement of foveal light reflex, retinal striae and thickening with membranous tissue in more advanced cases (Figure 1-4A)

Testing

- Amsler grid: distortion of lines with waviness, slanting, or bending
- OCT: reflective material on superficial retina with wrinkling or flattening of macular contour, retinal thickening, cystoid or schisis changes (Figure 1-4B)
- FA: can show hyperfluorescence indicating leakage from edema due to the traction exerted on retinal vessels

Differential Diagnosis

Macular edema, vitreomacular traction (VMT), lamellar macular hole

Management

- No treatment indicated when patient is asymptomatic, but continued semi-annual or annual monitoring is advised to detect progression
- PPV with membrane peeling; internal limiting membrane (ILM) peeling is optional and studies have shown mixed results in terms of effect on vision and recurrence rate. It is particularly effective for patients with significant metamorphopsia.

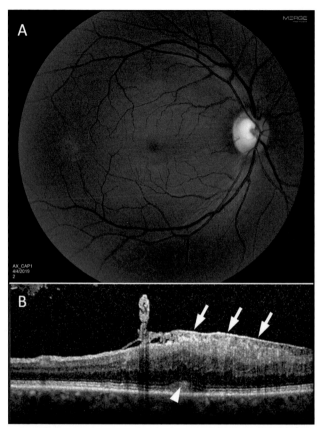

Figure 1-4. (A) Fundus photograph of a right eye with retinal striae due to an ERM. (B) OCT of a left eye with irregular macular contour, thickening, subfoveal ellipsoid zone disruption (arrowhead), and hyperreflective signal on inner surface (arrows) consistent with an ERM.

FULL-THICKNESS MACULAR HOLE

M. Ali Khan, MD

- Foveal defect involving all neural retinal layers, spanning from ILM to RPE
- Most cases are idiopathic (due to abnormal vitreo-foveal traction); secondary causes include trauma and pathologic myopia
- Prevalence: Ranges from 0.2 to 3.3 in 1000. Risk factors: female gender and older age (sixth decade of life or greater).
- Classification systems
  - Gass classification (exam-based, not imaging based): Stage 1 (impending hole), Stage 2 (small, < 400 μm defect), Stage 3 (large, > 400 μm defect), Stage 4 (full defect with associated complete posterior vitreous detachment)
  - International Vitreomacular Traction Study Group (IVTS)[9] classification (spectral domain-OCT [SD-OCT] based system). Full-thickness macular hole are classified by the following:
    - Size based on minimum hole diameter: small (≤ 250 um), medium (> 250 but ≤ 400 um), or large (> 400 um)
    - Status of vitreous: with or without VMT

Signs and Symptoms

Decreased central vision, metamorphopsia, and/or a central blind spot (scotoma); vision: near normal to severely reduced depending on size and duration

Exam Findings

Round, red-based appearing lesion at foveal center (Figure 1-5A), concurrent epiretinal membrane (ERM) may be

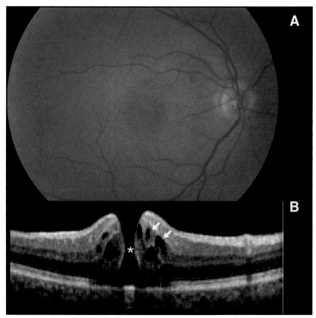

Figure 1-5. (A) A 74-year-old phakic patient with full-thickness macular hole. A round, red appearing foveal lesion was present. (B) SD-OCT revealed a full-thickness defect (*) with local pseudocysts (arrows).

present, Watzke-Allen sign: patient's description of discontinuity in center of thin slit beam centered over hole on fundoscopy

Testing

OCT: current standard for diagnosis shows a full-thickness defect from ILM to RPE seen on at least one B-scan image; hole width (in microns) is measured at narrowest linear hole diameter; hole edges often appear rounded and may have cystic changes (Figure 1-5B)

Differential Diagnosis

ERM with pseudohole, lamellar macular hole, cystoid macular edema (CME), outer retinal pathologies (solar retinopathy, alkyl nitrate ["popper"] related maculopathy)

Management

- Treatment options
  - Vitrectomy surgery (most common method of repair) with single surgery anatomic closure of hole is typically achieved in ~90% of initial cases. ILM peeling has been associated with improved hole closure rates and lower rates of reopening. Face-down positioning is common, though requirement and duration of positioning is a subject of debate; additional surgical maneuvers (use of silicone oil, ILM flaps, etc.) may be utilized in special cases.
  - Pharmacologic vitreolysis with intravitreal ocriplasmin
    - Microplasmin for Intravitreal Injection—Traction Release without Surgical Treatment (MIVI-TRUST) studies[10] revealed improved macular hole closure rates with ocriplasmin vs vehicle injection (40.6% vs 10.6%, $P < .001$). Smaller hole size was strongly associated with treatment success.
  - Pneumatic vitreolysis: Intravitreal injection of air or gas bubble. Small retrospective series have noted closure rates for small macular holes between 50% to 100%. Further data is necessary to refine rates. Available data suggests improved results with longer acting (C3F8) gas.
- Larger size and longer duration are associated with poor outcomes and observation may be appropriate in chronic cases with poor prognosis.

VITREOMACULAR TRACTION

M. Ali Khan, MD

Characterized by abnormal vitreous adhesion to the macula resulting in anatomic distortion of fovea. The anatomic alteration differentiates VMT from vitreomacular adhesion (VMA).

- Classification system
  - IVT classification[9] (SD-OCT based system)
    - All of the following 3 features must be present on at least one B-scan ultrasound: (1) partial perifoveal vitreous detachment, (2) vitreous adhesion to macula within a 3-mm radius of fovea, (3) associated distortion of the fovea but without full-thickness defect
    - VMT can be further categorized by size of VMA (focal [≤ 1500 μm] or broad [> 1500 μm]) and presence or absence of concurrent macular disease

Signs and Symptoms

Decreased central vision, metamorphopsia, and/or a central blind spot (scotoma)

Exam Findings

Macular schisis, subretinal fluid, and cystic changes; concurrent ERM and other macular disease may be present

Testing

- OCT: standard for diagnosis with IVTS classification system; features such as loss of foveal contour, macular schisis, subretinal fluid, and pseudocysts may be present (Figure 1-6)

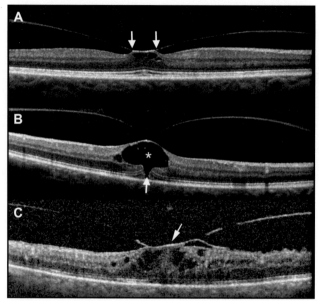

Figure 1-6. Representative examples of VMT. (A) Mild VMT demonstrating adhesion of the vitreous to the central macula (arrows) with edema limited to the inner retina. (B) More extensive foveal abnormality may be present, however, with larger cystic formation (*) and outer retinal disruption (arrow). (C) Concurrent ERM (arrow) with broad VMT may be present.

Differential Diagnosis

ERM with pseudohole, lamellar or full-thickness macular hole, CME, outer retinal pathologies (eg, solar retinopathy, alkyl nitrate ["popper"] related maculopathy)

Management

- Observation: spontaneous VMT release may be observed in 30% to 40% of eyes. Eyes with good presenting visual acuity and mild foveal changes may be monitored.

- Vitrectomy surgery: Single surgery anatomic release of VMT is typically achieved in >90% of cases. ILM peeling is common.
- Pharmacologic vitreolysis with FDA-approved intravitreal ocriplasmin (Jetrea)
  - Factors associated with resolution: age <65 years old, VMT adhesion diameter ≤1500 μm, phakic status, and absence of ERM were factors associated with resolution of VMT in post-hoc analysis
  - The Ocriplasmin for Treatment for Symptomatic Vitreomacular Adhesion Including Macular Hole (OASIS) study data revealed improved nonsurgical release of VMT in eyes treated with ocriplasmin compared to vehicle injection (41.7% vs 6.2%, *P* < .01)[11]
- Pneumatic vitreolysis

Cystoid Macular Edema

Ehsan Rahimy, MD

- Retinal thickening in macula due to disruption of blood-retinal barrier, resulting in fluid leakage from perifoveal capillaries into intracellular spaces of the retina
- Most commonly occurs following cataract surgery (between 1% to 3% of patients), known as pseudophakic CME or Irvine-Gass syndrome, typically several weeks after surgery

Signs and Symptoms

Decreased central vision, metamorphopsia, and/or photophobia

Exam Findings

Cysts in macula, sometimes in a petaloid configuration, with loss of foveal light reflex; depending on etiology, other retinal findings may be present (eg, retinal hemorrhages with venous tortuosity in retinal vein occlusion, or optic disc edema with or without vitreous cells in inflammatory causes)

Testing

- FA: In later phases of angiogram (5 to 15 minutes), leakage of dye into cystoid spaces is appreciated as hyperfluorescence emanating radially in Henle's layer, forming the classic "petaloid" leakage pattern (Figure 1-7A). May see staining and leakage from a "hot" optic nerve as well (eg, pseudophakic CME/Irvine-Gass syndrome).
- OCT: useful for detecting intraretinal fluid and contributing tractional forces such as ERM or VMT (Figure 1-7B)

Differential Diagnosis

DEPRIVEN is a common mnemonic device:

Diabetes

E2 prostaglandin analogues

Pars planitis and other intermediate/posterior uveitis

Retinitis pigmentosa (RP)

Irvine-Gass syndrome

Venous occlusion

Epinehprine

Niacin toxicity

Causes of non-leaking CME (no leakage on FA): retinitis pigmentosa (some types), Goldmann-Favre syndrome, niacin toxicity, taxanes, juvenile X-linked retinoschisis, tractional CME (eg, from ERM or VMT syndrome)

Management

- Depends on underlying cause

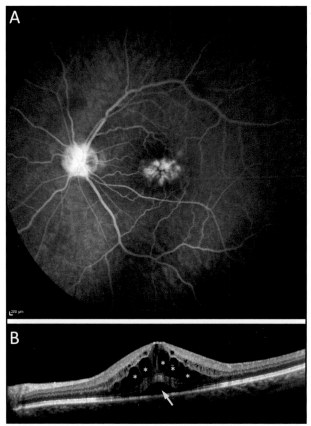

Figure 1-7. (A) FA demonstrating late angiographic edema in a petaloid distribution with associated optic disc staining in a patient with CME after cataract surgery. (B) OCT demonstrating CME (*) with concurrent subretinal fluid (arrow).

- Topical corticosteroids +/- nonsteroidal anti-inflammatory drugs work well for post-operative cases of CME (eg, Irvine-Gass syndrome)
- Topical (eg, dorzolamide) or systemic carbonic anhydrase inhibitors (eg, acetazolamide) for CME associated with RP and other inherited retinal degenerations
- Periocular, intravitreal, or systemic corticosteroids: preferable for cases not optimally controlled or responsive to topical therapy
- VEGF inhibitors: reduce vascular permeability from disrupted endothelium
- Vitrectomy: may be helpful in cases refractory to medical therapy (eg, chronic uveitis), or in those where a tractional component needs to be addressed (eg, release of posterior hyaloid, VMT, or ERM)

MYOPIC DEGENERATION

Mohamed K. Soliman, MD, MSc and
Michael Dollin, MD, FRCSC

- Characteristic degenerative changes occurring in a subset of patients with high myopia (refractive error ≥ -6.00 diopter or axial length ≥ 26 mm) as a result of progressive and excessive elongation of the globe
- Prevalence varies between 0.2% to 3.0% depending on age and ethnicity
- Longer axial length and increased age are significant risk factors

Signs and Symptoms

Asymptomatic in early stages, decreased vision, metamorphopsia, and scotoma from secondary complications

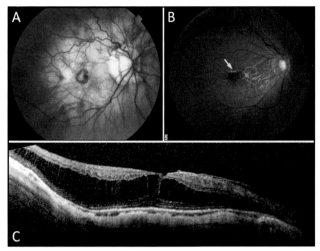

Figure 1-8. Myopic degeneration. (A) Color fundus photo with a Fuchs spot, demonstrating subfoveal hyperpigmentation. (B) Color fundus photo showing lacquer cracks (arrow). (C) OCT revealing myopic foveoschisis with large outer retinal cystic spaces.

Exam Findings

Posterior staphyloma (PS): focal outpouching of sclera typically involving posterior pole; chorioretinal atrophy: RPE attenuation resulting in visible underlying choroidal vessels early on and patchy or diffuse atrophy in posterior pole and periphery later; Fuchs spot: small patch of RPE hyperplasia that follows regressed CNV (Figure 1-8A); lacquer cracks: yellow, irregular, subretinal streaks in posterior pole from breaks in Bruch's membrane may lead to CNV (Figure 1-8B); anomalous optic disc: may be small, large or tilted with crescent-shaped peripapillary chorioretinal atrophy; other signs: vitreous syneresis, dome-shaped macula (DSM), peripapillary intra-choroidal cavitation; associated complications include CNV (5% to 10%), foveoschisis (9% to

33%), macular hole, retinal breaks, and rhegmatogenous retinal detachment

Testing

- OCT: presence of CNV, foveoschisis, macular hole, PS, and DSM (Figure 1-8C)
- FA: window defect in areas of RPE atrophy and lacquer cracks, focal hyperfluorescence with subtle leakage in CNV, hypofluorescence in areas of hyperpigmentation or hemorrhage
- B-scan ultrasonography: presence of staphyloma

Differential Diagnosis

Neovascular AMD, dystrophies such as choroideremia, gyrate atrophy, and generalized choroidal dystrophy, presumed ocular histoplasmosis, tilted optic disc syndrome

Management

Treatments aimed at slowing myopia progression in children include low-dose (0.01%) topical atropine sulfate and increasing daily exposure to outdoor sunlight

Treatment of Myopic Choroidal Neovascularization

Anti-VEGF agents typically achieve control with 1 to 4 injections, however, CNV may recur in at least 10% of cases.

Treatment of Myopic Foveoschisis

- Observation, if the patient is relatively asymptomatic
- Surgical management
  - Optimal timing is controversial, but proposed indications include visual decline, severe and progressive foveoschisis, macular detachment, and macular hole formation

- Pars plana vitrectomy (PPV) with or without ILM peeling and gas tamponade to relieve tractional forces at the vitreoretinal interface
- Macular buckling to relieve external tractional forces from progressive globe elongation and PS, more commonly performed outside the United States

ANGIOID STREAKS

Alok S. Bansal, MD

- Crack-like dehiscences in Bruch's membrane associated with multiple systemic conditions, vulnerable to subretinal hemorrhage from minor blunt trauma
- Most common systemic conditions include pseudoxanthoma elasticum (PXE), Ehlers-Danlos, Paget's disease, sickle cell disease, or idiopathic (Use PEPSI as a mnemonic device).

Signs and Symptoms

Asymptomatic, metamorphopsia and/or vision loss from CNV

Exam Findings

Reddish-brown bands radiating from optic nerve (Figure 1-9), typically bilateral, subretinal hemorrhage if CNV or choroidal rupture, if associated with PXE, fundus may show a mottled appearance in temporal macula ("peau d'orange") and optic nerve drusen

Testing

- Lab workup depends on suspected underlying systemic condition: PXE (skin biopsy and/or *ABCC6* gene mutation), Paget's disease (elevated serum alkaline phosphatase), sickle cell hemoglobin electrophoresis

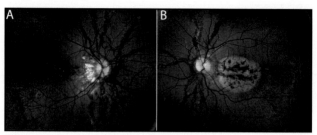

Figure 1-9. (A) Color fundus photo of right eye showing classic reddish-brown bands radiating from optic nerve that characterize angioid streaks. (B) Color fundus photo of left eye showing macular atrophy secondary to prior subretinal hemorrhage in addition to the angioid streaks.

- OCT: may show intraretinal and/or subretinal fluid if CNV
- Fluorescein angiogram: confirm presence of CNV
- Dermatologic evaluation: small, yellow papular lesions on neck with skin laxity characteristic of PXE (Figure 1-10)

Differential Diagnosis

AMD, pathologic myopia (lacquer cracks), ocular histoplasmosis syndrome, choroidal rupture

Management

- Observation with periodic examination if no signs of CNV; intravitreal anti-VEGF injections if (+) CNV
- Management of underlying systemic condition with internist
- Strict eye protection due to risk of hemorrhage from minor trauma

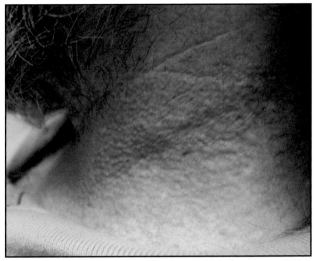

Figure 1-10. Raised yellow bumps on lateral neck that are characteristic of PXE.

POLYPOIDAL CHOROIDAL VASCULOPATHY

Ehsan Rahimy, MD

Demographics: typically > 60 years old, men > women with predilection for Asian and African ethnicity

Signs and Symptoms

Blurred vision, metamorphopsia, and central/paracentral scotoma if significant hemorrhage

Exam Findings

Orange/red nodular structures with aneurysmal dilations (polyps) beneath RPE; may be associated with serous PED, neurosensory serous detachment, and lipid exudates; classic presentation:

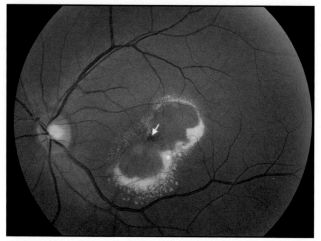

Figure 1-11. Color fundus photograph showing juxtafoveal polyps (arrow) with associated retinal hemorrhage and lipid exudation (*).

subretinal hemorrhage and/or hemorrhagic PED which may be large (Figure 1-11)

Testing

- OCT: useful for detecting subretinal and/or sub-RPE fluid, PEDs, and even polyps (dome-like RPE elevations with moderate internal reflectivity)
- FA: polypoidal lesions may resemble occult choroidal neovascular membranes demonstrating hyperfluorescence due to leakage; associated hemorrhage would show up as an area of hypofluorescence due to blockage (Figure 1-12)
- Indocyanine green angiography: differentiates polypoidal choroidal vasculopathy from other forms of neovascularization, as it reveals a branching network of polyps in the choroid (see Figure 1-12)

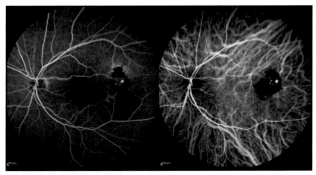

Figure 1-12. Fluorescein (left) and indocyanine green (right) angiography demonstrates the blocking effect (hypofluorescence/hypocyanescence) of hemorrhage surrounding focal hyperfluorescence/hypercyanescence consistent with a polypoidal lesion.

Differential Diagnosis

Neovascular AMD, myopic CNV, chronic central serous retinopathy with associated CNV

Management

- Intravitreal injections of VEGF inhibitors, PDT, or combination of both. Polypoidal choroidal vasculopathy is particularly responsive to PDT compared to classic wet AMD.[12]
- Surgical vitrectomy: evacuate significant breakthrough vitreous hemorrhage or to displace significant submacular hemorrhage

CENTRAL SEROUS CHORIORETINOPATHY

John D. Pitcher III, MD

- Sub-neurosensory retina fluid accumulation from choroidal source
- Young and middle-aged adults with a male predominance
- Etiology is not fully understood. An association has been made with psychological stress and Type A personalities, which may be a surrogate for elevated endogenous corticosteroid. Also associated with pregnancy, obstructive sleep apnea, systemic corticosteroid and exogenous testosterone exposure.

Signs and Symptoms

Asymptomatic if central fovea not affected, blurred vision, metamorphopsia, micropsia, blind spot, decreased color vision

Exam Findings

Serous retinal detachment (Figure 1-13A), RPE detachment, in chronic cases, subretinal fluid may "gutter" inferiorly and may cause RPE atrophy

Testing

- OCT: subretinal fluid (Figure 1-13C), RPE detachment, choroidal thickening (best visualized with enhanced depth imaging) in affected and fellow eye (Figure 1-14)
- OCT angiography: noninvasive detection of CNV
- FA: Early focal hyperfluorescence with late leakage and pooling (Figure 1-13B) or less commonly, a "smoke stack" appearance; choroidal neovascular membrane will show more diffuse leakage. Chronic disease may have window defects from RPE atrophy, as well as more diffuse or multi-focal leakage with possible "guttering" inferiorly.

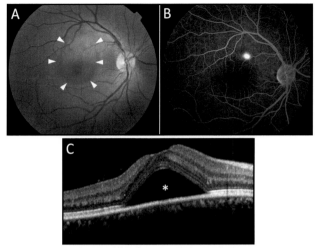

Figure 1-13. (A) Color photograph in a patient with acute central serous chorioretinopathy shows a circular, well-defined area of retinal elevation (arrowheads). (B) FA shows focal late leakage. (C) Spectral domain-OCT shows subretinal fluid (*) involving the fovea which resolved 3 months after onset.

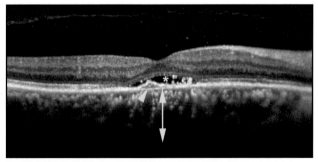

Figure 1-14. Spectral domain-OCT in a patient with chronic central serous chorioretinopathy shows an RPE detachment (arrowhead) with adjacent subretinal fluid (*). Choroidal thickening (double arrow) is also evident.

- Indocyanine green angiography: zones of transient choroidal vascular permeability, hot spots of leakage

Differential Diagnosis

CNV, AMD, polypoidal choroidal vasculopathy, hypertensive choroidopathy, Vogt-Koyanagi-Harada disease, posterior scleritis, optic pit maculopathy

Management

- Cessation of corticosteroid (and androgen) exposure, in coordination with medical provider
- Acute: observation for spontaneous resolution in most cases
- Chronic: PDT has most evidence for efficacy; focal laser photocoagulation may be considered for extra-foveal disease; other options include intravitreal anti-VEGF injections, oral eplerenone, spironolactone, or mifepristone although evidence of efficacy is limited
- Consideration for workup and treatment of obstructive sleep apnea

OPTIC DISC PIT MACULOPATHY

Allen Chiang, MD

- Congenital optic pit arises from incomplete closure of embryonic fissure
- Rare (1/10,000) with no known risk factors. Usually unilateral (80% to 90%) with associated serous macular detachment in 25% to 75% of cases.

Signs and Symptoms

Decreased vision, metamorphopsia, micropsia, scotoma if there is associated macular detachment

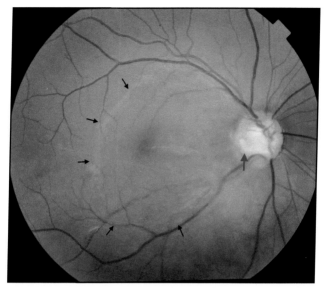

Figure 1-15. Optic disc pit located at temporal margin of the disc (blue arrow) with associated serous macular detachment (black arrows).

Exam Findings

Pit is usually located at temporal aspect of nerve as a depression that differs in color from surrounding tissue, but may be situated anywhere along the margin or centrally; serous retinal detachment or retinoschisis may extend from the pit (Figure 1-15)

Testing

- Perimetry: enlarged blind spot and/or relative central scotoma
- Amsler grid: distortion corresponding to area of edema and/or subretinal fluid

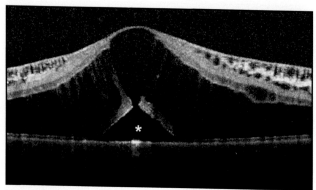

Figure 1-16. OCT scan of ODP-M highlights the presence of subretinal fluid (*) and severe retinoschisis.

- OCT: identifies the pit and any subretinal fluid or retinoschisis, particularly on a radial scan through the optic nerve and nasal macula (Figure 1-16)
- FA: unremarkable with no leakage of dye in the serous detachment

Differential Diagnosis

Optic nerve abnormalities (eg, coloboma), tilted optic disc syndrome, peripapillary staphyloma, optic nerve hypoplasia, glaucoma, central serous retinopathy; CNV

Management

- No treatment indicated for isolated optic pit without maculopathy
- Regular monitoring (eye exams and Amsler grid testing) to detect optic disc pit maculopathy (ODP-M). Once present, prolonged observation is associated with poor visual outcomes and is not advisable.
- Treatment options for ODP-M

- ○ Laser photocoagulation to form a barricade between the pit and serous detachment is noninvasive, but of variable success
- ○ PPV with gas tamponade: remove vitreous traction and redirect fluid away from the macula

CHOROIDAL FOLDS

Eugene A. Milder, MD

Indentation of the inner surface of the sclera relative to the choroid results in parallel folds of the choroid, RPE, and retina

Signs and Symptoms

Decreased vision, metamorphopsia, may be asymptomatic

Exam Findings

Parallel, alternating lighter and darker bands deep to the retina usually in and around the posterior pole; not typically seen in the periphery (Figure 1-17A)

Testing

- OCT: demonstrates folding of the choroid, RPE and retina (Figure 1-17B)
- FA: highlights the choroidal folds due to hyperfluorescence at the crests of the folds, hypofluorescence in the troughs
- Fundus autofluorescence: enhances the appearance of choroidal folds
- B-scan ultrasound: can identify choroidal pathology such as choroidal thickening and a T-sign due to posterior scleritis
- Orbital imaging (using computed tomography [CT] or magnetic resonance imaging [MRI]): if orbital pathology such as an intraorbital tumor is suspected

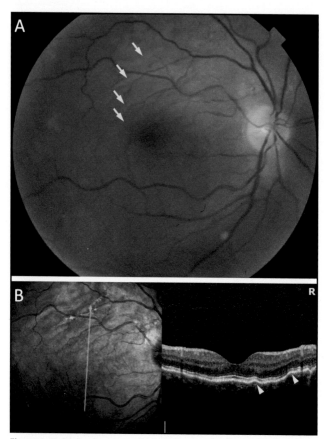

Figure 1-17. (A) Fundus photo of idiopathic macular choroidal folds (arrows). (B) Corresponding OCT showing undulation of the choroid, retinal pigment epithelium, and outer retina (arrowheads).

Differential Diagnosis

Idiopathic (most common) and hyperopia is often present; a helpful mnemonic is THIN RPE: tumors, hypotony, idiopathic and inflammation, neovascular membrane, retrobulbar mass, papilledema, and extraocular hardware (eg, scleral buckle)

Management

- No treatment is indicated for idiopathic choroidal folds.
- For secondary choroidal folds, identifying the etiology is critical since treatment may be warranted depending on the underlying cause.

HYPOTONY MACULOPATHY

Eugene A. Milder, MD

- Distortion of macular anatomy due to low intraocular pressure (IOP), often defined as <5 mmHg. Often part of hypotony syndrome which includes corneal decompensation, accelerated cataract formation, and discomfort.
- Common etiologies include surgery (eg, over-filtering blebs from glaucoma surgery), inflammation, or trauma (eg, cyclodialysis cleft).
- Most cases typically present unilaterally. However, bilateral cases may arise from systemic conditions such as uremia, dehydration, acidosis.

Signs and Symptoms

Decreased vision and metamorphopsia, asymptomatic in mild cases, discomfort and/or pain may be present in the setting of hypotony syndrome

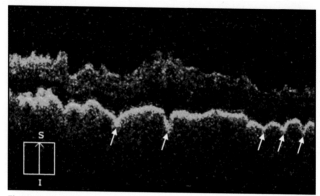

Figure 1-18. OCT demonstrating full-thickness chorioretinal folds (arrows) in hypotony maculopathy.

Exam Findings

Chorioretinal folds in the macula (Figure 1-18), vascular tortuosity, other ocular features of hypotony may also be present: choroidal swelling or detachment in the periphery, optic nerve edema, corneal edema/folds, shallow or flat anterior chamber

Testing

- OCT: macular chorioretinal folds, increased choroidal thickness
- FA: enhances the appearance of chorioretinal folds due to hyperfluorescence at the crests of the folds, hypofluorescence in the troughs
- B-scan ultrasound: increased choroidal thickness, serous choroidal detachment
- Anterior segment OCT or ultrasound biomicroscopy (UBM) may be helpful if the cause of hypotony is unclear (eg, cyclodialysis cleft)

Differential Diagnosis

Idiopathic choroidal folds (often associated with hyperopia), posterior scleritis, orbital mass or inflammation, CNV

Management

- Treatment varies depending on underlying etiology, but aim is to normalize IOP. For example, over filtering blebs can be treated with pressure patches, cessation of topical steroid, or surgical revision. Cyclodialysis clefts can be repaired surgically.

- Associated serous choroidal detachments will usually resolve as IOP improves and can be treated with corticosteroids and cycloplegic drops. If appositional, surgical drainage is indicated. Vision recovery is often delayed and/or incomplete, especially in cases of prolonged hypotony.

REFERENCES

1. Age-Related Eye Disease Study Research Group. A randomized, placebo-controlled, clinical trial of high-dose supplementation with vitamins C and E, beta carotene, and zinc for age-related macular degeneration and vision loss: AREDS report no. 8. *Arch Ophthalmol.* 2001;119(10):1417-1436. doi:10.1001/archopht.119.10.1417

2. Age-Related Eye Disease Study 2 Research Group. Lutein + zeaxanthin and omega-3 fatty acids for age-related macular degeneration: the Age-Related Eye Disease Study 2 (AREDS2) randomized clinical trial. *JAMA.* 2013;309(19):2005-2015. doi:10.1001/jama.2013.4997

3. Brown DM, Michels M, Kaiser PK, Heier JS, Sy JP, Ianchulev T; ANCHOR Study Group. Ranibizumab versus verteporfin photodynamic therapy for neovascular age-related macular degeneration: two-year results of the ANCHOR study. *Ophthalmology.* 2009;116(1):57-65.e5. doi:10.1016/j.ophtha.2008.10.018

4. Rosenfeld PJ, Brown DM, Heier JS, et al; MARINA Study Group. Ranibizumab for neovascular age-related macular degeneration. *N Engl J Med.* 2006;355(14):1419-1431. doi:10.1056/NEJMoa054481

5. Martin DF, Maguire MG, Fine SL, et al. Comparison of Age-related macular Degeneration Treatments Trials (CATT) Research Group. Ranibizumab and bevacizumab for treatment of neovascular age related macular degeneration:two-year results. *Ophthalmology.* 2012;119(7):1388-1398.doi:10.1016/j.ophtha.2012.03.053

6. Heier JS, Brown DM, Chong V, et al; VIEW 1 and VIEW 2 Study Groups. Intravitreal aflibercept (VEGF trap-eye) in wet age-related macular degeneration. *Ophthalmology.* 2012;119(12):2537-2548. doi:10.1016/j.ophtha.2012.09.006

7. Dugel PU, Koh A, Ogura Y, et al. HAWK and HARRIER Study Investigators. HAWK and HARRIER: Phase 3, Multicenter, Randomized, Double-Masked Trials of Brolucizumab for Neovascular Age-Related Macular Degeneration. *Ophthalmology.* 2020;127(1):72-84.

8. Gragoudas ES, Adamis AP, Cunningham ET Jr, Feinsod M, Guyer DR; VEGF Inhibition Study in Ocular Neovascularization Clinical Trial Group. Pegaptanib for neovascular age-related macular degeneration. *N Engl J Med.* 2004;351(27):2805-2816. doi:10.1056/NEJMoa042760

9. Duker JS, Kaiser PK, Binder S, et al. The International Vitreomacular Traction Study Group classification of vitreomacular adhesion, traction, and macular hole. *Ophthalmology.* 2013;120(12):2611-2619. doi:10.1016/j.ophtha.2013.07.042

10. Stalmans P, Benz MS, Gandorfer A, et al; MIVI-TRUST Study Group. Enzymatic vitreolysis with ocriplasmin for vitreomacular traction and macular holes. *N Engl J Med.* 2012;367(7):606-615. doi:10.1056/NEJMoa1110823

11. Dugel PU, Tolentino M, Feiner L, Kozma P, Leroy A. Results of the 2-Year Ocriplasmin for Treatment for Symptomatic Vitreomacular Adhesion Including Macular Hole (OASIS) Randomized Trial. *Ophthalmology.* 2016;123(10):2232-2247. doi:10.1016/j.ophtha.2016.06.043

12. Koh A, Lee WK, Chen LJ, et al. EVEREST study: efficacy and safety of verteporfin photodynamic therapy in combination with ranibizumab or alone versus ranibizumab monotherapy in patients with symptomatic macular polypoidal choroidal vasculopathy. *Retina.* 2012;32(8):1453-1464. doi:10.1097/IAE.0b013e31824f91e8

2

Retinal Vascular Diseases

NONPROLIFERATIVE DIABETIC RETINOPATHY

Sasha Hubschman, MD and
Jayanth Sridhar, MD

- Hyperglycemia results in endothelial damage in retinal capillaries, leading to vascular remodeling, leakage, and occlusion.
- Twenty-three percent of people with type 1 diabetes mellitus develop diabetic retinopathy (DR) after 5 years, 80% after 15 years. Up to 21% of patients with type 2 diabetes mellitus already have retinopathy at time of initial diagnosis of diabetes.
- Intense glycemic control is associated with reduced progression to severe nonproliferative diabetic retinopathy (NPDR) and proliferative diabetic retinopathy (PDR).

Hsu J, Chiang A, eds. *The Pocket Guide to Medical Retina* (pp 39-79).
© 2021 Taylor & Francis Group.

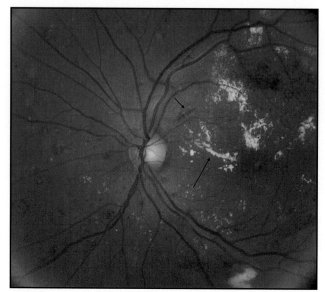

Figure 2-1. NPDR with intraretinal hemorrhages (short arrow) and exudates (long arrow).

Signs and Symptoms

Blurred vision, usually due to presence of macular edema (see the Diabetic Macular Edema section) or, less commonly, from macular ischemia

Exam Findings

- Mild NPDR (5% risk of progression to PDR in 1 year): >1 microaneurysm, criteria not met for other levels of DR
- Moderate NPDR (15% risk of progression to PDR in 1 year): hemorrhage/microaneurysm (Figure 2-1) or soft exudates (cotton wool spots [CWS]), venous beading that do not meet criteria for severe NPDR

- Severe NPDR (52% risk of progression to PDR in 1 year): 4:2:1 rule; hemorrhage/microaneurysm in all 4 quadrants or venous beading in ≥ 2 quadrants or intraretinal microvascular abnormalities (IRMA) in at least 1 quadrant
- Diabetic macular edema (DME): may arise at any stage

Testing

- Systemic: fasting blood glucose, hemoglobin A1C every 3 months; check blood pressure; blood test for hyperlipidemia if extensive exudate is present
- Optical coherence tomography (OCT): evaluate for presence and severity of DME
- Fluorescein angiography (FA): identify areas of ischemia, leakage from microaneurysms, and neovascularization (Figure 2-2)
- Optical coherence tomography angiography (OCTA): dyeless alternative to FA to assess severity of retinopathy (microaneurysms, capillary non-perfusion, etc; Figure 2-3)

Differential Diagnosis

Branch or central retinal vein occlusion (CRVO), ocular ischemic syndrome, hypertensive retinopathy, radiation retinopathy

Management

- Tight glycemic, blood pressure, and lipid control regardless of stage
- Regular follow-up is crucial to assess for progression of disease
    - In type 1 diabetics: Initial exam 5 years after onset, then annually if retinopathy present. Frequency of follow-up based on previous retinal exam and A1C level. Optimal screening intervals range from months in patients with severe NPDR to every year for those without retinopathy.

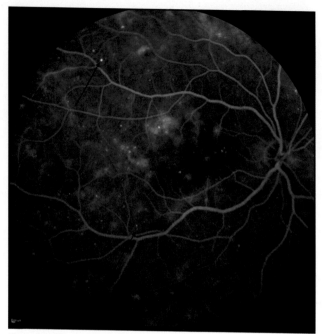

Figure 2-2. FA can demonstrate microaneurysms (arrows) in NPDR.

- ○ In type 2 diabetics: Initial exam upon diagnosis and then annually. More frequent screening may be necessary based on stage of NPDR.
- Pregnancy poses higher risk of developing worsening retinopathy and patient should be examined during first trimester and followed closely until 1 year post-partum. Vitreous surgery, intravitreal corticosteroids, and laser therapy are safe during pregnancy. No randomized controlled trials to prove safety of anti-VEGF during pregnancy and is therefore generally avoided.

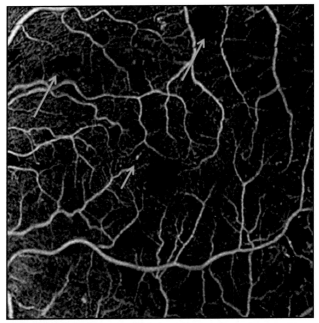

Figure 2-3. OCTA of the superficial plexus (6×6 mm) reveals areas of non-perfusion (long arrows) as well as microaneurysmal changes (short arrow).

- Mild and moderate NPDR: generally not treated unless DME is present
- Severe or very severe NPDR and patients with higher risk of progressing to PDR: May consider anti-VEGF therapy to reduce retinopathy severity and rate of progression even in absence of DME. Panretinal photocoagulation may also be considered, particularly if there is heightened concern for non-compliance with recommended follow-up.

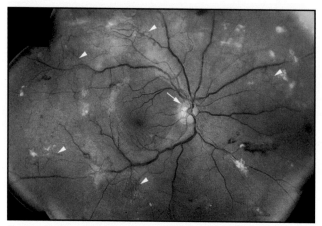

Figure 2-4. PDR with NVD (arrow) and elsewhere (arrowheads).

PROLIFERATIVE DIABETIC RETINOPATHY

Michael J. Venincasa, MD and
Jayanth Sridhar, MD

- PDR is the leading cause of vision loss in working-age Americans.
- Prevalence ↑ with duration of diabetes mellitus. Other risk factors include hypertension, smoking, nephropathy, dyslipidemia, and pregnancy.
- Pathophysiology: diabetic microvascular changes → retinal ischemia → increased angiogenic growth factors → secondary neovascularization (Figure 2-4) → complications (eg, vitreous hemorrhage [VH], tractional retinal detachment [TRD])

Signs and Symptoms

Many are initially asymptomatic; blurred vision, floaters, shadows, pain if intraocular pressure (IOP) is elevated

Exam Findings

- Stages of PDR
  - Early: neovascularization is present, but does not meet high-risk criteria
  - High-risk: (1) neovascularization of the optic disc (NVD) ≥ 1/3 to 1/2 disc area, or (2) NVD and vitreous or pre-retinal hemorrhage, or (3) neovascularization elsewhere (NVE) ≥ 1/2 disc area and VH or preretinal hemorrhage
  - Severe: posterior fundus obscured by VH or preretinal hemorrhage or macula center detached
- Macular edema can be present at any stage of PDR and should be addressed concomitantly (see the Diabetic Macular Edema section)

Testing

- FA: although PDR can be diagnosed on exam, FA (particularly wide-field FA) is helpful to identify retinal ischemia and capillary non-perfusion, leakage from neovascularization, and can often show more than is readily apparent on clinical examination
- OCT: can assist with assessment of macular edema and monitoring for progression to macular involvement in cases with TRD (Figure 2-5)
- Other testing: HbA1C, lipid profile, blood pressure

Differential Diagnosis

Radiation retinopathy, branch retinal vein occlusion (BRVO)/CRVO, macular telangiectasia, retinal vasculitis, sarcoidosis, ocular ischemic syndrome, sickle cell retinopathy

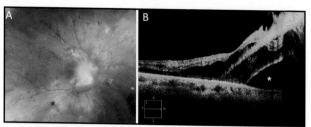

Figure 2-5. PDR complicated by (A) TRD confirmed with subretinal fluid (*) visible in the macula on (B) OCT.

Management

- Good glycemic and blood pressure control can reduce risk of PDR progression

- Panretinal Photocoagulation (PRP): mainstay of treatment for decades that reduces retinal response to hypoxia, induces regression of neovascularization, and based on the Diabetic Retinopathy Study, reduces vision loss by 50%[1]

- Intravitreal anti-VEGF therapy

  ○ A Phase 3 clinical trial[2] found this noninferior to PRP for PDR in terms of visual acuity. Secondary outcomes including visual field loss and rates of vitrectomy favored anti-VEGF therapy slightly over PRP.

  ○ First-line treatment for DME, so this is increasingly favored as initial therapy in patients with both DME and PDR

  ○ If utilized as monotherapy, patient compliance to the follow-up and treatment schedule is critical as the treatment effect is not durable like PRP.

- Pars plana vitrectomy (PPV) surgery is indicated for dense or non-clearing VH and macula-involving TRD.

- Glaucoma filtering surgery may be indicated if there is angle closure due to neovascularization.

Diabetic Macular Edema

Jordan D. Deaner, MD and
Carl D. Regillo, MD

- Common manifestation of DR that reduces central vision and is the leading cause of vision loss in developed world
- Etiology: Chronic hyperglycemia leads to breakdown in the blood-retinal barrier (maintained by pericytes and endothelial cell tight junctions) and increased vasopermeability (mediated by VEGF).

Signs and Symptoms

Decreased vision, metamorphopsia

Exam Findings

- Slit lamp biomicroscopy: thickening (edema) of macula with or without cystoid changes centrally, microaneurysms, and lipid exudation
- Clinically significant macular edema (CSME) as defined by Early Treatment Diabetic Retinopathy Study (ETDRS; Figure 2-6)[3]
  - Retinal thickening within 500 μm of center of the fovea
  - Hard exudate with adjacent retinal thickening at or within 500 μm of center of the macula
  - Retinal thickening 1 disc area or larger, any part of which is within 1 disc diameter of center of macula

Testing

- OCT: shows retinal thickening typically with cystic change and subretinal fluid when severe (Figure 2-7)
  - Allows quantification of degree and location (central vs non-central) of edema

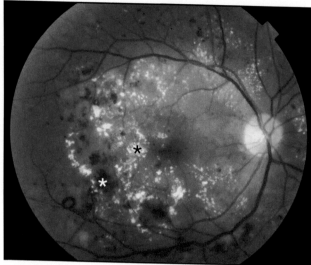

Figure 2-6. Color fundus photograph demonstrating CSME, hard exudates (black *), and retinal hemorrhages (white *) in severe NPDR.

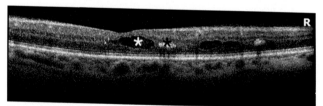

Figure 2-7. OCT shows mild cystic macular edema (white *) and hard exudates (black *) in the central macula of a patient with DME and moderate NPDR.

- ○ Reveals associated vitreoretinal interface abnormalities, such as epiretinal membrane (ERM) or vitreomacular traction (VMT)
- ○ Useful for monitoring response to therapy

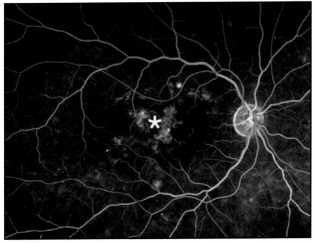

Figure 2-8. Intravenous FA demonstrating numerous microaneurysms and late macular leakage (*) in a patient with severe NPDR and DME.

- FA: reveals leakage from incompetent capillaries or microaneurysms along with other features of DR (Figure 2-8)
- OCTA: noninvasive alternative to FA shows status of macular perfusion and can rule out other pathology such as choroidal neovascularization (Figure 2-9)
- Miscellaneous: blood glucose, hemoglobin A1c (HbA1c), lipid panel, blood pressure

Differential Diagnosis

Post-operative cystoid macular edema (Irvine-Gass syndrome), cystoid macular edema from medications (epinephrine, E2-prostaglandins, nicotinic acid), retinal vein occlusion (RVO), choroidal neovascularization, hypertensive retinopathy, ocular ischemic syndrome, radiation retinopathy, retinal arterial macroaneurysm; uveitis

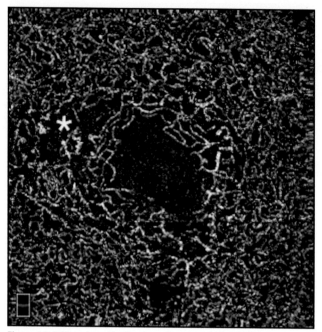

Figure 2-9. OCT angiography showing enlargement of the foveal avascular zone and focal loss of the deep vascular plexus (*) in a patient with DME.

Management

- Asymptomatic patients with mild and/or non–center-involving macular edema may initially be observed.
- Intravitreal anti-VEGF agents are first-line therapy for center-involving (CI) DME.
    - Ranibizumab and aflibercept are approved by the Food and Drug Administration (FDA) for treating DME.
    - Bevacizumab is used off-label.

- Results of DRCR Network Protocol T[4] show that afliber-cept, bevacizumab, and ranibizumab all improved vision and decreased macular thickness.
    - Worse presenting visual acuity (< 20/40): Aflibercept group had greater degree of vision improvement at 1 year compared to other agents. At 2 years, no significant difference between ranibizumab and aflibercept.
    - Both on-label drugs had either better visual outcomes or better reduction in DME at 2 years compared with bevacizumab in eyes with more severe DME at presentation (Table 2-1)
- Corticosteroids (intravitreal triamcinolone, dexamethasone implant, fluocinolone implant) are generally considered to be second-line therapy for CI DME
    - Longer-lasting than anti-VEGF agents: up to 3 to 4 months for intravitreal triamcinolone and dexamethasone implant; 2 to 3 years for fluocinolone implant
    - Often used when there is inadequate response to anti-VEGF agents or as an alternative to ongoing, frequent anti-VEGF injections
    - Side effects: IOP elevation and cataract progression
- Focal macular laser photocoagulation: proven in ETDRS[3] to decrease risk of vision loss in eyes with CSME, but inferior to anti-VEGF or corticosteroids (DRCR Network Protocol I[5]) as far as improving vision in eyes with CI DME
    - May be considered for non-CI DME that has not completely responded to intravitreal pharmacotherapy
- PPV and membrane peeling may be considered if vitreo-macular interface abnormalities are contributing to macular edema, particularly if response to medical treatment is suboptimal.

Table 2-1. Protocol T: Comparison of Average Visual Acuity Gain in Letters Between Aflibercept, Bevacizumab, and Ranibizumab at 1 and 2 Year Follow-Up

| | AVERAGE VISUAL ACUITY GAIN (LETTERS) | | | |
| | *1 Year Follow-Up* | | *2 Year Follow-Up* | |
	Equal to or better than 20/40	Worse than 20/40	Equal to or better than 20/40	Worse than 20/40
Aflibercept	8.0	18.9*	7.8	18.3*
Bevacizumab	7.5	11.8	6.8	13.3
Ranibizumab	8.3	14.2*	8.6	16.1
Significance	Not significantly different	P < .05 for aflibercept and ranibizumab vs bevacizumab	Not significantly different	P < .05 for aflibercept vs bevacizumab
* Statistically significant				

Cotton Wool Spots

Ashley Khalili, MD and
David Y. Rhee, MD

- Represent focal areas of nerve fiber layer ischemia and thrombosis of the precapillary arteriole, resulting in swelling of ganglion cell axons due to interrupted axoplasmic flow (Figure 2-10)
- Histopathology: hallmark finding of cytoid bodies within the CWS, which are eosinophilic segments of ganglion cell axons that are dilated due to interrupted axoplasmic flow and accumulation of intracellular material

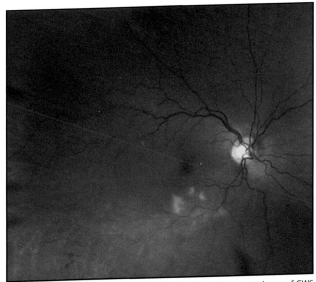

Figure 2-10. A patient with inferior BRVO occlusion with a sectoral area of CWS on color fundus photography.

Signs and Symptoms

Often asymptomatic unless there is foveal involvement, occasionally scotoma or vague description of blurred vision, systemic symptoms of an underlying etiology may be present

Exam Findings

Focal white or yellow-white, slightly elevated and fluffy lesions in the superficial retina, usually smaller than 1/3 disc areas in diameter and most commonly in the posterior pole; usually disappear within 4 to 12 weeks, but may last longer in diabetes.

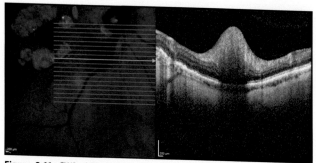

Figure 2-11. CWS. OCT of the CWS with localized retinal nerve fiber layer thickening.

Testing

- OCT: focal retinal nerve fiber layer thickening and hyper-reflectivity in the inner retina (Figure 2-11)
- FA: may reveal areas of capillary non-perfusion near CWS

Associated Systemic Conditions

DR, RVO, retinal artery occlusion (RAO), acute malignant hypertensive retinopathy; HIV/AIDS: associated with a low CD4 count (noninfectious), anemia, bacteremia or fungemia; embolic process: fat embolism syndrome, carotid or cardiac emboli, endocarditis; leukemia/lymphoma; immune/inflammatory disorders and collagen vascular disease: systemic lupus erythematosus, polyarteritis nodosa, giant cell arteritis, dermatomyositis, scleroderma; shaken baby syndrome (less common finding, retinal hemorrhages are more common); Purtscher and Purtscher-like retinopathy, radiation retinopathy, ocular ischemic syndrome

Differential Diagnosis

Hard exudate, retinal infiltrate, drusen, chorioretinal atrophy, chorioretinitis, myelinated nerve fiber layer

Management

- Treatment is directed to addressing the underlying condition
- Presence of even a single CWS requires a workup to determine etiology including:
  - Workup for undiagnosed diabetes or hypertension (a single CWS can be the earliest ophthalmoscopic finding of either condition)
  - If no underlying systemic condition is identified, further workup with PCP for systemic vascular conditions is warranted.
    - Recommended tests: complete blood count, HIV screen, basic chemistry
    - Additional studies may be warranted depending on review of symptoms: echocardiography, carotid ultrasound, and serology to workup collagen vascular disease

HYPERTENSIVE RETINOPATHY

Shilpa Gulati, MD, MS and
David Y. Rhee, MD

- Systemic hypertension (systolic blood pressure > 140 mmHg and diastolic > 90 mmHg) leads to acute and chronic changes in the retina, choroid, and optic nerve
- Risk factors: African American ethnicity, family history, obesity, high salt diet, and tobacco and alcohol use

Signs and Symptoms

Acute or malignant hypertension may present with headache and blurry vision; chronic changes may be asymptomatic

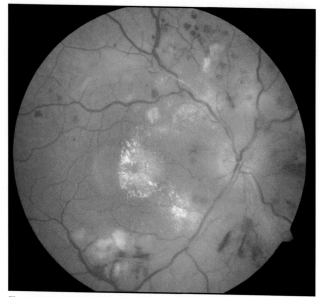

Figure 2-12. Fundus photo demonstrating grade 4 hypertensive retinopathy: optic nerve edema, serous retinal detachment, intraretinal hemorrhages, and CWS. (Reprinted with permission from Chirag P. Shah, MD, MPH.)

Exam Findings

- Acute or malignant hypertension (Figure 2-12): retinal hemorrhages (varied morphologies include sub-inner limiting membrane [ILM], intraretinal, and subretinal), CWS, subretinal fluid, optic disc edema; choroidal fibrinoid necrosis (choriocapillaris non-perfusion leading to ischemic necrosis of the retinal pigment epithelial [RPE]) appears as gray-yellow choroidal lesions which become hyperpigmented over time, resulting in Elschnig spots (if clustered) or Siegrist streaks (if linear)

- Chronic hypertension (Figure 2-13): arteriolar narrowing (artery to vein width ratio < 2:3), copper wiring, silver wiring

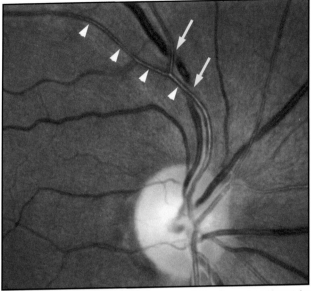

Figure 2-13. Fundus photo of arterio-venous nicking (arrows) and arteriolar copper wiring (arrowheads), hallmarks of chronic hypertensive retinopathy. (Reprinted with permission from William E. Benson, MD.)

(narrowed artery with no visible blood flow within walls), hardened arteries compressing veins within their common adventitial sheath causes arterio-venous nicking (Gunn sign) or deflection of veins at the crossing (Salus sign)

- Scheie classification is a commonly used grading scale: (1) mild arteriolar narrowing, (2) arteriolar narrowing with focal vessel irregularity, (3) grade 2 with exudates or hemorrhage, (4) grade 3 with optic disc edema

Testing

Measurement of systolic and diastolic blood pressure

Differential Diagnosis

DR, radiation retinopathy, RAO, blood dyscrasias, juxtafoveal telangiectasia, vasculitis, ocular ischemic syndrome

Management

- Further workup if a secondary systemic condition is suspected: renal artery stenosis, pre-eclampsia, pheochromocytoma, primary hyperaldosteronism, Cushing's syndrome, coarctation of the aorta, obstructive sleep apnea, hyperparathyroidism, and hyperthyroidism
- Hemoglobin A1c measurement in diabetic patients
- Optimization of diet and blood pressure via primary care providers
- Emergency or inpatient management in cases of symptomatic acute or malignant hypertension. Admission is indicated for blood pressure > 180/120 with end-organ damage, including optic disc edema, given high-risk of morbidity and mortality without prompt treatment.

RETINAL ARTERY OCCLUSION

Phoebe L. Mellen, MD and
Ferhina S. Ali, MD, MPH

- Compromised blood flow within the retinal arterial system due to thromboembolism, vasospasm, or an inflammatory process
- Variable sites of involvement: central retinal artery (CRAO), superior and inferior branches of CRA, branch retinal artery (BRAO), cilioretinal artery
- Risk factors: age, male gender, smoking, diabetes, hypertension, hyperlipidemia, systemic coagulopathy

Signs and Symptoms

Sudden painless vision loss or transient graying of vision, complete scotoma (CRAO) or sectoral scotoma (BRAO), relative afferent pupillary defect

Exam Findings

Retinal whitening in area of retinal ischemia, distal thinning and boxcarring of blood vessels, cherry red spot (fovea), embolic material within blood vessel lumen (eg, Hollenhorst plaque) (Figures 2-14A and 2-14B)

Testing

- FA: delayed arterial filling distal to the location of the occlusion, delayed arterio-venous transit time (see Figure 2-14B). Delayed choroidal filling suggests ophthalmic artery or carotid disease.
- OCT: inner retinal hyperreflectivity and thickening in the area of ischemia (acute), inner retinal thinning and atrophy (chronic; Figure 2-14C)
- Electroretinogram: diminished b-wave (reflects inner retinal ischemia)
- Laboratory workup (URGENT)
    - \> 50 years old and no embolus seen on exam: must consider giant cell arteritis and obtain CBC, ESR/CRP
    - < 50 years old: hyperocoagulability workup
    - Full stroke evaluation (Magnetic resonance imaging [MRI]/magnetic resonance angiogram [MRA] brain scan, carotid ultrasound vs MRA of the neck, electrocardiogram, echocardiogram)

Differential Diagnosis

Cherry red spot (Tay-Sachs disease, lysosomal storage diseases); retinal whitening due to infectious causes (eg, acute retinal

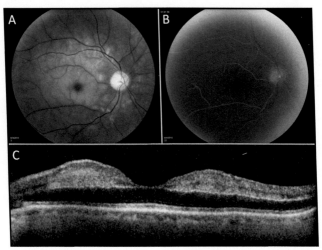

Figure 2-14. (A) Fundus photograph of CRAO with retinal whitening and cherry red spot along with attenuation and boxcarring of arterioles. (B) Early arterial phase of fluorescein angiogram shows both delayed arterial filling and arteriovenous transit. (C) Spectral domain-OCT of the macula with inner retinal thickening and hyperreflectivity consistent with acute ischemia.

necrosis [ARN]; progressive outer retinal necrosis [PORN], syphilis); ischemic vasculopathy (diabetes mellitus, sickle retinopathy, vasculitis [lyme, sarcoid])

Management

- Ocular emergency in acute cases! Refer urgently for stroke evaluation.
- Ocular massage/anterior chamber paracentesis: historically this was suggested to possibly help dislodge an embolus, but clinical efficacy remains unproven
- Carbogen therapy (combination of carbon dioxide and oxygen) to dilate vasculature has been attempted but clinical efficacy is also unproven

- Tissue plasminogen activator not recommended for RAO due to side effects of administration (intracranial hemorrhage) and unproven vision benefit
- If neovascularization develops, treatment is with anti-VEGF therapy and PRP laser
- Associated neovascular glaucoma may require glaucoma surgery
- Visual prognosis depends on degree of ischemia and is usually poor in CRAO. If a cilioretinal artery is present, there may be some sparing of macular blood flow and some visual recovery.
- Sectoral field loss in BRAO is usually permanent

RETINAL VEIN OCCLUSION

Katherine E. Talcott, MD

- Common retinal vascular abnormality caused by thrombus in central retinal vein near lamina cribrosa (CRVO) or arterio-venous crossing point (BRVO). Complications: macular edema, retinal ischemia, neovascularization leading to glaucoma, VH and/or retinal traction.
- Typically unilateral in patients > 50 years old. Systemic risk factors for CRVO: hypertension, open angle glaucoma and diabetes mellitus; for BRVO: hypertension, cardiovascular disease, open angle glaucoma, high body mass index.

Signs and Symptoms

Sudden painless loss of vision or visual field defect; may be asymptomatic if more peripheral or if occlusion is mild; floaters from VH, typically due to neovascularization

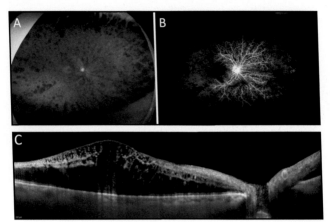

Figure 2-15. (A) Wide-field imaging of an ischemic CRVO. (B) Wide-field FA demonstrates severe macular ischemia and peripheral non-perfusion. (C) OCT demonstrates severe intraretinal macular edema. (Reprinted with permission from Christopher M. Aderman, MD.)

Exam Findings

- CRVO: retinal hemorrhages (superficial flame shaped and deep blot) in all 4 quadrants ("blood and thunder" appearance), dilated and tortuous retinal veins (Figure 2-15A); other findings: optic nerve swelling, CWS, macular edema, neovascularization (iris, angle, retinal) or VH, optociliary shunt (collateral) vessels
- BRVO: wedge-shaped distribution of intraretinal hemorrhage based on location of venous blockage; most common location is superotemporal arcade (Figure 2-16A)

Testing

- FA: delayed filling of occluded retinal vein; capillary non-perfusion (non-perfused CRVO has ≥ 10 disc areas of retinal capillary non-perfusion), microaneurysms, telangiectatic collateral vessels, leakage from macular edema or

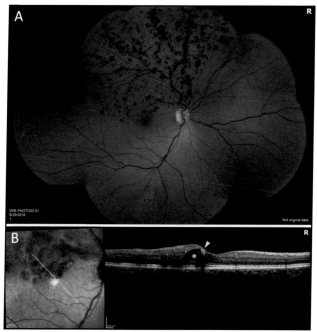

Figure 2-16. (A) Fundus photograph of a superotemporal BRVO. (B) OCT shows intraretinal edema (*) and hemorrhage (arrowhead).

retinal neovascularization; chronic cases may only reveal microvascular changes after hemorrhages have resolved (Figure 2-15B)

- OCT: may show cystoid edema, subretinal fluid, and/or photoreceptor loss from longstanding macula edema or ischemia (Figures 2-15C and 2-16B)
- OCTA: reduction of blood vessel density, mainly of deep capillary plexus

Differential Diagnosis

DR, ocular ischemic syndrome, hypertensive retinopathy, blood dyscrasias, radiation retinopathy

Management

- No treatment is available to reverse RVO. The goal is to manage secondary macula edema and/or neovascularization.
- Medical therapy
  - ○ VEGF therapy is considered first-line treatment for associated macular edema, providing significant gains in visual acuity and decreased edema.[6,7] Also useful for inducing regression of iris and retinal neovascularization. Ranibizumab and aflibercept are FDA-approved. Bevacizumab is off-label.
  - ○ Steroid agents
    - Intravitreal triamcinolone acetonide: beneficial for macular edema due to CRVO but does not demonstrate benefit for BRVO
    - Steroid implants: also used to treat macular edema, dexamethasone implant is FDA-approved
- Focal/grid laser photocoagulation: second-line treatment for BRVO as adjunct to anti-VEGF or steroids; no visual benefit for CRVO
- Laser PRP: Used for iris and retinal neovascularization in CRVO. Sectoral application in area of occlusion is indicated for neovascularization in BRVO.
- For atypical presentations (bilateral/recurrent RVO, younger patients without cardiovascular risk factors), rule out inflammatory or hypercoagulable conditions

OCULAR ISCHEMIC SYNDROME

Samuel K. Steven Houston III, MD

- Chronic ocular hypoperfusion secondary to carotid stenosis >90% from atherosclerosis; usually unilateral and affects both anterior and posterior segment
- Risk factors: hypertension, diabetes, ischemic cardiac or cerebrovascular disease, peripheral vascular disease

Signs and Symptoms

Subacute or acute vision loss; less commonly, transient vision loss (amaurosis fugax); variable visual field defects; pain may be ischemic or due to increased IOP and may be lessened by supine position (ocular angina)

Exam Findings

- Anterior segment: corneal edema, episcleral injection, flare and cell, poorly reactive pupil with iris and angle neovascularization, asymmetric cataract
- Posterior segment: dilated (but not tortuous) retinal veins, narrowing of arterioles, mid-peripheral round blot retinal hemorrhages (classic finding), NVD or elsewhere (NVE; Figure 2-17)

Testing

- Check blood pressure
- Emergent evaluation of carotid arteries: carotid Doppler, computed tomography angiogram, MRA
  - Carotid evaluation often shows ipsilateral stenosis >90%
- Fluorescein angiogram: delayed choroidal filling; delayed arterio-venous transit, mid-peripheral hemorrhages; mid-peripheral ischemia; late vascular leakage (Figure 2-18)

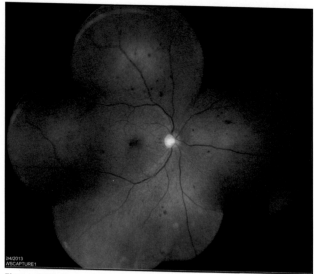

Figure 2-17. Ocular ischemic syndrome. Color fundus photo with mainly mid-peripheral hemorrhages. Note the veins are slightly dilated but not tortuous and the arterioles are very attenuated. (Reprinted with permission from Michael Dollin, MD, FRCSC.)

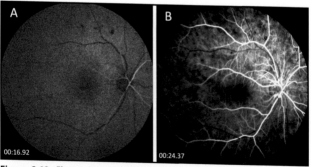

Figure 2-18. Fluorescein angiogram demonstrating delayed arterio-venous transit time characteristic of ocular ischemic syndrome with partial filling of the arterioles early (A) and complete filling occurring over 7 seconds later (B). (Reprinted with permission from Michael Dollin, MD, FRCSC.)

Differential Diagnosis

CRVO, DR, hypertensive retinopathy

Management

- Emergent evaluation of carotids and consultation with vascular surgeon, if needed
- Topical steroid and cycloplegic for anterior segment inflammation
- Neovascularization: anti-VEGF injection followed by panretinal photocoagulation may reduce risk of neovascular glaucoma
- Medical treatment of increased IOP but if (+) neovascular glaucoma, surgical treatment (eg, aqueous shunt implant) or diode laser cyclophotocoagulation

RETINAL ARTERY MACROANEURYSM

Durga S. Borkar, MD and
Allen Chiang, MD

- Incidence is approximately 1 case per 9000 eyes
- Older age and hypertension are risk factors; approximately 10% are bilateral

Signs and Symptoms

Often asymptomatic; vision loss may be noted secondary to macular edema or hemorrhage; metamorphopsia or decreased vision can be reported with macular involvement; floaters due to VH

Exam Findings

Most common location for a symptomatic macroaneurysm is along the superotemporal arcade; typically, an outpouching of

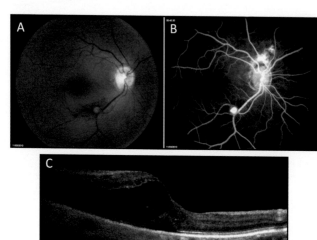

Figure 2-19. Multimodal imaging panel consisting of (A) color fundus photography of a retinal artery macroaneurysm along the inferior arcade with associated intraretinal hemorrhage, (B) fluorescein angiogram of the same eye with pooling within the macroaneurysm, and (C) OCT (vertical section) with associated macular edema and subfoveal fluid.

arterial wall may be visible, but due to hemorrhage or exudation, imaging may be necessary to confirm diagnosis (Figure 2-19A)

Testing

- FA: macroaneurysm will appear as a round, focal area of pooling. Later phases may show leakage which can be helpful in guiding treatment (Figure 2-19B).
- OCT: quantifies both exudates and macular edema (Figure 2-19C)

Differential Diagnosis

Coats disease, Von Hippel-Lindau syndrome, BRVO, DR, radiation retinopathy

Management

- Workup for systemic hypertension and possibly systemic vascular disease
- Consider focal laser to leaking aneurysms when central macula is involved or threatened
- Anti-VEGF is typically not effective in the treatment of macular edema secondary to a leaking or ruptured retinal artery macroaneurysm.

MACULAR TELANGIECTASIA

*Thomas Jenkins, MD and
Jason Hsu, MD*

- Type 1 (aneurysmal telangiectasia): typically unilateral congenital vascular abnormality that primarily affects males and is considered a variant of Coats disease; no systemic disease associations
- Type 2 (perifoveal telangiectasia): bilateral and typically occurs in fourth to sixth decade with a reported prevalence of < 0.1%; variable outcomes depending on degree of macular atrophy or the development of subretinal neovascularization (SRNV); frequently associated with diabetes mellitus

Signs and Symptoms

Type 1: unilateral decreased vision; Type 2: blurred paracentral vision and metamorphopsia; frequently good visual acuity at presentation (eg, ~20/30); worse visual acuity with development of SRNV or central foveal atrophy

Exam Findings

- Type 1: telangiectatic vessels in the temporal or nasal macula; capillary, venular, and arteriolar aneurysms of variable

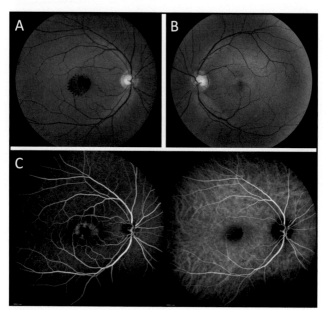

Figure 2-20. (A) Color photograph of the right eye with newly diagnosed proliferative macular telangiectasia type 2 demonstrating subretinal and intraretinal hemorrhage affecting the fovea. (B) Color photograph of the left eye of same patient with signs of nonproliferative disease with telangiectatic venules, gray discoloration of the parafovea, and refractile superficial deposits. (C) Fluorescein angiogram (left) and indocyanine green (right) imaging pair of the right eye demonstrating leakage from overlying telangiectatic vessels with blockage of the underlying subretinal neovascular membrane by hemorrhage. The indocyanine green angiogram demonstrates right angle venules.

size; exudates and macular edema frequently present; vascular changes may be present in the peripheral fundus

- Type 2: grayish discoloration with loss of temporal parafoveal transparency; superficial refractile retinal deposits without exudation; telangiectatic vasculature, blunted right angle venules; stellate plaques of RPE hypertrophy; proliferative form associated with SRNV with associated exudation (Figures 2-20A and 2-20B)

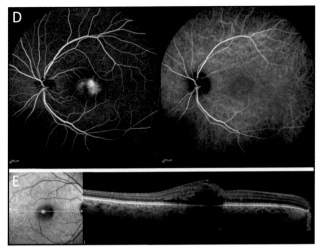

Figure 2-20 (continued). (D) FA of the left eye shows leakage that spares the central fovea despite the absence of neovascularization. Indocyanine green in the left eye is unremarkable. (E) OCT of the right eye showing subretinal and intraretinal hemorrhage and edema.

Testing

- Type 1
  - ○ FA: Early demonstration of telangiectatic macular vessels with microaneurysms of variable size with late associated leakage. Patchy areas of capillary non-perfusion may be present.
  - ○ OCT: Intraretinal cystoid macular edema with retinal thickening and intraretinal hard exudates. Subretinal fluid may be present (Figure 2-20E).
  - ○ OCTA: Decreased macular capillary density around telangiectatic vessels in the superficial and deep capillary plexus. Focal capillary dilation in the deep capillary plexus.

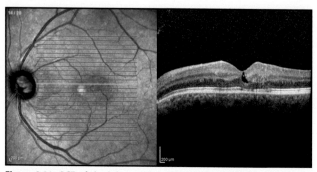

Figure 2-21. OCT of the left eye of a patient with nonproliferative macular telangiectasia type 2 showing temporal parafoveal hyporeflective intraretinal spaces representing neurodegeneration with disruption of the ellipsoid layer.

- Type 2
  - FA: early demonstration of parafoveal telangiectatic vessels with subsequent leakage in temporal parafoveal macula without extension into central fovea (Figures 2-20C and 2-20D)
  - OCT: Classic finding is intraretinal cystoid-like hyporeflective spaces with ellipsoid zone/RPE disruption just temporal to the fovea (Figure 2-21). ILM drape may also be observed. Intraretinal pigment migration in advanced cases; subretinal fluid and hemorrhage above the retinal pigment epithelium if SRNV is present (Figure 2-20E).
  - OCTA: Decreased parafoveal vascular density in the superficial and deep vascular plexus with dilation and telangiectasia of existing vessels. Neovascularization in the outer retina if SRNV is present.
  - Fundus autofluorescence (FAF): relative hyperautofluorescence due to loss of foveal luteal pigment

Differential Diagnosis

DR, age-related macular degeneration, RVO, radiation retinopathy, sickle cell retinopathy, lamellar macular hole, Coats disease

Management

- No treatment is consistently effective for macular telangiectasia type 1.
  - There may be a role for anti-VEGF, steroids or laser in some patients.
- No treatment is currently indicated for macular telangiectasia type 2 in the absence of neovascularization. With evidence of SRNV, anti-VEGF injections may be beneficial.

SICKLE CELL RETINOPATHY

Travis J. Peck, MD and
Carl H. Park, MD

- Sickle cell disease is a group of inherited red blood cell disorders
- Sickle cell trait found in 8% of African-Americans, rare in other ethnicities
- Compound heterozygotes for the mutation (Hb SC) more likely to develop retinopathy than homozygotes (Hb SS)

Signs and Symptoms

Ranging from asymptomatic to severe loss of vision, floaters and flashes

Exam Findings

Goldberg Stages of Retinopathy

- Stage I: peripheral arterial occlusions; Stage II: peripheral arterio-venous anastomoses; Stage III: preretinal neovascularization; Stage IV: VH; Stage V: retinal detachment

Classic Findings in Sickle Cell

- Nonproliferative: superficial retinal hemorrhages in periphery that appear as round salmon patches progressing to black sunburst spots; angioid streaks (Figure 2-22A)
- Proliferative: primarily peripheral neovascularization with white sea fan appearance; tractional and rhegmatogenous retinal detachments

Testing

- Hemoglobin electrophoresis for sickle cell disease
- Wide-field FA: peripheral sea fan neovascularization posterior to capillary non-perfusion (Figure 2-22B)
- OCT: inner retinal atrophy sparing photoreceptor layer and retinal pigment epithelium

Differential Diagnosis

DR, retinal vascular occlusion, hypertensive retinopathy, ocular ischemic syndrome, familial exudative vitreoretinopathy, Eales disease

Management

- Nonproliferative disease may be observed with exam every 6 months
- Anit-VEGF injection or laser photocoagulation anterior to border of non-perfused and perfused retina for proliferative disease

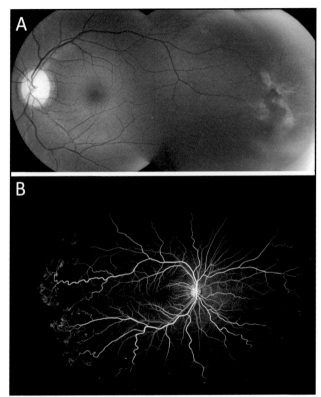

Figure 2-22. (A) Peripheral salmon patch of preretinal hemorrhage representing peripheral neovascularization in sickle cell retinopathy. (B) Wide-field FA with severe peripheral non-perfusion and leakage from sea fan neovascularization.

- For select cases (with good follow-up adherence), areas of neovascular process may be observed to make sure it does not progress, as the area may auto-infarct
- Vitrectomy for non-clearing VH and retinal detachment

Radiation Retinopathy

Shilpa Gulati, MD, MS and
David C. Reed, MD

- Chronic and progressive microangiopathy that may follow exposure to plaque brachytherapy or charged particle radiotherapy (eg, external beam radiation, proton beam, or gamma knife). Loss of retinal capillary endothelial cells (sparing pericytes) leads to vascular permeability, occlusion, non-perfusion, and ischemia.

- Delayed onset with peak incidence at 2 to 3 years; can arise as early as 4 months after treatment. Radiation maculopathy has been reported in 10% to 63% of eyes following plaque for choroidal melanoma, with proliferative disease in 3% to 25% of eyes.

Risk Factors

- Comorbid diabetes, hypertension, and pregnancy; concurrent chemotherapy
- Dose-dependent: generally requires > 35 Gy of total radiation
- Tumor characteristics: height, basal diameter, and location relative to fovea
- Mode of delivery: shielding of ocular structures from external beam radiation may decrease radiation to the macula
- Fraction size: hyperfractionation is associated with decreased incidence

Signs and Symptoms

Early stages of retinopathy may be asymptomatic; patients may present with blurry vision or floaters

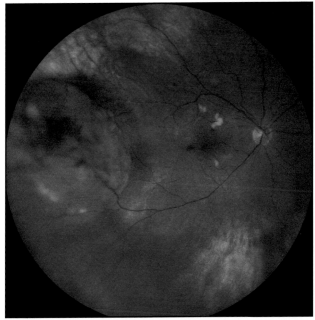

Figure 2-23. Radiation retinopathy. Fundus photo taken 10 months after I-125 plaque brachytherapy for choroidal melanoma, showing CWS, intraretinal hemorrhages, and exudate. (Reprinted with permission from Jay S. Duker, MD.)

Exam Findings

Telangiectasia, microaneurysms, intraretinal hemorrhages, CWS, lipid exudates, macular edema, vascular sheathing (Figure 2-23). Proliferative disease: retinal/optic nerve/anterior segment neovascularization, VH, TRD, neovascular glaucoma.

Testing

- OCT: evaluate for macular edema (Figure 2-24A)
- FA: demonstrates microaneurysms, focal capillary closure, ischemia, and leakage from proliferative disease

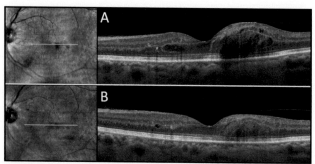

Figure 2-24. (A) Macular OCT showing perifoveal intraretinal fluid in a patient with a history of plaque brachytherapy for choroidal melanoma. Visual acuity is 20/50. (B) Following intravitreal bevacizumab, there is reduction in the intraretinal fluid and an improvement in vision to 20/40. (Reprinted with permission from Jay S. Duker, MD.)

Differential Diagnosis

DR, hypertensive retinopathy; retinal artery or vein occlusion, Coats disease, macular telangiectasia, ocular ischemic syndrome

Management

- Prevention: not widely practiced; periocular triamcinolone at the time of plaque application, or early laser photocoagulation to the expected area of ischemia around the tumor base, may decrease incidence or severity of maculopathy

- Macular edema: Case series have demonstrated transient improvement in macular edema with intravitreal bevacizumab (Figure 2-24B), intravitreal triamcinolone, and focal/grid laser photocoagulation; however, impact on visual acuity is modest and repeat injections are often needed to sustain improvement.

- Proliferative disease: sectoral or PRP is indicated for retinal, optic nerve, or anterior segment neovascularization; PPV for non-clearing VH or TRD

- Enucleation may be indicated in cases complicated by neovascular glaucoma.
- Case reports exist of successful treatment with photodynamic therapy, hyperbaric oxygen, and oral pentoxifylline.

REFERENCES

1. The Diabetic Retinopathy Study Research Group. Preliminary report on effects of photocoagulation therapy. *Am J Ophthalmol*. 1976;81(4):383-396. doi:10.1016/0002-9394(76)90292-0

2. Gross JG, Glassman AR, Liu D, et al; Diabetic Retinopathy Clinical Research Network. Five-Year Outcomes of Panretinal Photocoagulation vs Intravitreous Ranibizumab for Proliferative Diabetic Retinopathy: A Randomized Clinical Trial. *JAMA Ophthalmol*. 2018;136(10):1138-1148. doi:10.1001/jamaophthalmol.2018.3255

3. Early Treatment Diabetic Retinopathy Study Research Group. Photocoagulation for diabetic macular edema. Early Treatment Diabetic Retinopathy Study report number *Arch Ophthalmol*. 1985;103(12):1796-1806. doi:10.1001/archopht.1985.01050120030015

4. Wells JA, Glassman AR, Ayala AR, et al; Diabetic Retinopathy Clinical Research Network. Aflibercept, bevacizumab, or ranibizumab for diabetic macular edema. *N Engl J Med*. 2015;372(13):1193-1203. doi:10.1056/NEJMoa1414264

5. Elman MJ, Bressler NM, Qin H, et al. Expanded 2-year follow-up of ranibizumab plus prompt or deferred laser or triamcinolone plus prompt laser for diabetic macular edema. *Ophthalmology*. 2011;118(4):609-614.

6. Varma R, Bressler NM, Suñer I, et al; BRAVO and CRUISE Study Groups. Improved vision-related function after ranibizumab for macular edema after retinal vein occlusion: results from the BRAVO and CRUISE trials. *Ophthalmology*. 2012;119(10):2108-2118. doi:10.1016/j.ophtha.2012.05.017

7. Heier JS, Clark WL, Boyer DS, et al. Intravitreal aflibercept injection for macular edema due to central retinal vein occlusion: two-year results from the COPERNICUS study. *Ophthalmology*. 2014;121(7):1414-1420.e1. doi:10.1016/j.ophtha.2014.01.027

3

Infectious Inflammatory Diseases

ENDOPHTHALMITIS

Meera D. Sivalingam, MD and
Sunir J. Garg, MD, FACS

- Inflammation of vitreous and aqueous, typically due to an infection
- Exogenous: most common type, categorized depending upon underlying cause
  - Acute post-operative: within 6 weeks of surgery, incidence after cataract surgery reported between 0.13% and 0.7% a year, incidence following pars plana vitrectomy (PPV) reported between 0.02% and 0.15%
  - Subacute post-operative: weeks to months after surgery, common pathogens include *Propionibacterium acnes, Staphylococcus*, fungi
  - Filtering bleb associated: may occur months to years after surgery, incidence between 0.12% and 1.2%

Hsu J, Chiang A, eds. *The Pocket Guide to Medical Retina* (pp 81-117).
© 2021 Taylor & Francis Group.

- ○ Post-trauma: days to weeks after penetrating trauma
- ○ Post-intravitreal injection: days after injection, reported incidence ranges in the literature but is approximately 0.05%
- Endogenous
  - ○ Bacterial: hematogenous seeding of the eye from bacteremia; 40% of cases occur in patients with endocarditis commonly caused by *Streptococcus* and *Staphylococcus* species; may occur in patients with urinary tract infections commonly caused by *Escherichia coli*; associated with intravenous drug abuse due to transient bacteremia commonly from *Bacillus cereus*
  - ○ Yeast: typically *Candida* species; found in patients who are immunocompromised, on long-term antibiotic treatment, or have indwelling catheters
  - ○ Fungal: rare in North America; may be exogenous or endogenous; *Aspergillus* and *Fusarium* are the most common pathogens; occurs in immunocompromised patients with persistent fungemia

Signs and Symptoms

Decreased vision, eye pain, red eye, floaters

Exam Findings

- Anterior segment: eyelid edema, conjunctival injection, corneal edema, anterior chamber cell, hypopyon, severe anterior chamber reaction with fibrin[1] (Figure 3-1)
- Posterior segment: vitreous cell, vitreous debris, decreased red reflex, retinal hemorrhages, retinal vascular sheathing, choroidal detachment (Figure 3-2)
- Pathogen dependent, ranges from focal chorioretinitis with low-grade vitritis to panophthalmitis

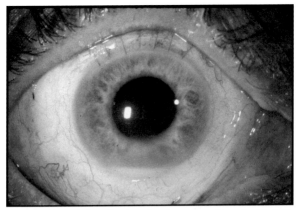

Figure 3-1. External photo showing subacute post-operative endophthalmitis with mild conjunctival injection, keratic precipitates, and hypopyon.

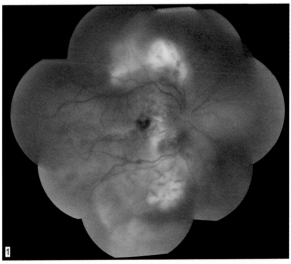

Figure 3-2. Color fundus photo of the right eye in the setting of methicillin-susceptible *Staphylococcus aureus* endogenous endophthalmitis showing vitritis, diffuse chorioretinitis, and retinal hemorrhages.

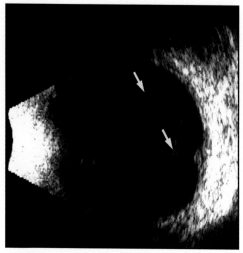

Figure 3-3. B-scan showing vitreous debris (arrows) and dense vitritis in an eye with post-operative endophthalmitis.

Testing

- Rule out wound/bleb leak, exposed suture
- B-scan if posterior view is limited: may reveal vitritis, choroidal thickening (Figure 3-3)
- Complete medical workup in endogenous infection

Differential Diagnosis

Acute noninfectious uveitis, sterile endophthalmitis, neoplastic conditions including retinoblastoma and lymphoma, retinochoroidal infection

Management

- Bacterial: Vitreous (or anterior chamber) tap sent for gram stain/culture with injection of intravitreal antibiotics. If endogenous, patients should undergo systemic workup to identify the source of infection and receive appropriate systemic antibiotics.

- Common intravitreal injection preparations: vancomycin (1 mg/0.1 ml) and ceftazidime (2.25 mg/0.1 ml); consider amikacin (0.4 mg/0.1 ml) instead of ceftazidime if allergic to penicillin/cephalosporins
- Endophthalmitis Vitrectomy Study (EVS): evaluated role of PPV and intravenous antibiotics in management of postcataract surgery bacterial endophthalmitis and found the following:
  - Systemic antibiotics did not improve visual outcomes
  - Hand motion or better vision: no difference in outcomes between immediate tap and inject vs PPV
  - Light perception vision: improved visual outcomes with immediate PPV
- Fungal and yeast: intravitreal voriconazole (0.1 mg/0.1 ml) or amphotericin (5 mcg/0.1 ml); vitrectomy with intravitreal injection

OCULAR TOXOPLASMOSIS

Nikolas J. S. London, MD

- Ubiquitous parasite/protozoa (*Toxoplasma gondii*), endemic in tropical environments. In North America, definitive host is the domestic cat.
- Most common etiology of posterior uveitis in immunocompetent patients
- Congenital (transplacental) infections typically involve the macula and may be bilateral; acquired (postnatal) infections are typically extramacular and unilateral

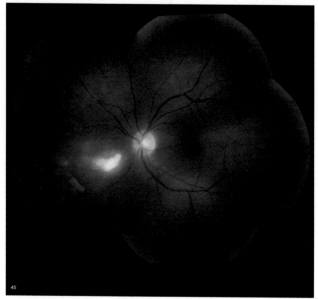

45

Figure 3-4. Color fundus photograph of the left eye shows a creamy yellow-white area of retinitis nasal to the optic disc and associated vasculitis with peri-arterial Kyrieleis plaques.

Signs and Symptoms

Systemic: acute infection is often asymptomatic, but may present with fever, malaise, sore throat, and/or lymphadenopathy in 10% to 20% of adults with acquired toxoplasmosis; Ocular: prominent blurred vision and floaters, often painless unless there is significant anterior uveitis

Exam Findings

- Creamy-yellow, circular area of retinitis with secondary involvement of choroid and sclera which is often adjacent to a chorioretinal scar (Figure 3-4), prominent vitritis

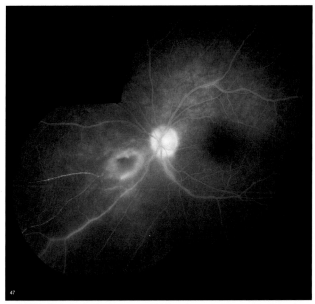

Figure 3-5. FA of the same eye seen in Figure 3-4 shows hyperfluorescence in the area of retinitis, adjacent perivascular staining and mild leakage, and optic disc staining.

("headlight-in-fog" appearance), vasculitis with possible peri-arterial exudates (Kyrieleis plaques), potential vascular occlusion; potential elevated intraocular pressure (IOP)

Testing

- Fluorescein angiography (FA): leakage in area of active lesion, perivascular staining and leakage, optic disc leakage (Figure 3-5)
- Serology for toxoplasmosis antibodies IgG and IgM. IgM indicative of acute infection and does not appear after repeated exposures. IgM does not cross the placental barrier while IgG does. IgG is indicative of previous exposure.

- Polymerase chain reaction (PCR) testing of ocular fluid (vitreous and/or aqueous) can be helpful in challenging cases
- Magnetic resonance imaging (MRI) scan of the brain in immunocompromised patients to assess central nervous system involvement

Differential Diagnosis

Necrotizing herpetic retinitis, syphilis, ocular tuberculosis, endogenous endophthalmitis, ocular lymphoma

Management

Treatment may not be necessary in all cases.
- Treatment criteria: macular or juxtapapillary lesion, lesions that threaten a large vessel, prominent hemorrhage, visual acuity impaired by 2 or more lines attributable to inflammation; immunocompromised patient
- Bactrim DS (trimethoprim-sulfamethoxazole) 800 mg/160 mg double-strength twice a day by mouth; pyrimethamine (100 mg loading dose followed by 25 to 50 mg once a day) and sulfadiazine (1 g 4 times a day) for 4 to 6 weeks. Give with folic acid (3 to 5 mg twice a week) to prevent leukopenia and thrombocytopenia; clindamycin 300 mg every 6 hours for 3 or more weeks; atovaquone 750 mg 4 times a day for 3 months.
- Topical cycloplegic and corticosteroid for significant anterior segment inflammation
- Systemic corticosteroids are often unnecessary unless threatening macula. If used, start 24 to 48 hours after initiation of antibiotics and taper prior to stopping antibiotics.

PRESUMED OCULAR HISTOPLASMOSIS SYNDROME

Katherine E. Talcott, MD

- Characterized by atrophic chorioretinal scars, peripapillary atrophy, and absence of intraocular inflammation that can lead to a choroidal neovascular membrane (CNV)
- May be due to infection with yeast form of *Histoplasma capsulatum*, a fungus endemic to the Ohio and Mississippi river valleys
- May also represent an inflammatory reaction triggered by certain organisms, including *H. capsulatum*, as disease is linked to human leukocyte antigen (HLA) haplotypes DRw2 and B7

Signs and Symptoms

Painless vision loss, metamorphopsia, and central/paracentral scotomas, due to CNV; often asymptomatic without CNV

Exam Findings

Characteristic (often bilateral) findings include: (1) discrete, atrophic or "punched-out" choroidal scars in macula or periphery, smaller in size than optic disc; confluent mid-peripheral scars in a linear or curvilinear pattern may be present (Figure 3-6A), (2) peripapillary atrophy, (3) absence of intraocular inflammation. Findings may be accompanied by a CNV (risk is 25% in patients with macular scars) that can progress to disciform scarring with subretinal fibrovascular tissue.

Testing

- FA: window defects of hyperfluorescence in areas of atrophy; CNV can be identified by leakage of fluorescein dye (Figure 3-6B)

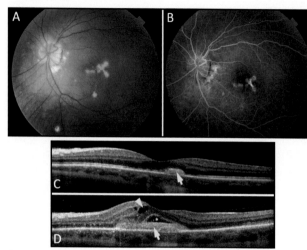

Figure 3-6. (A) Fundus photograph of left eye showing multiple chorioretinal scars and peripapillary atrophy consistent with presumed ocular histoplasmosis syndrome. (B) FA demonstrates window defects. (C) OCT shows subretinal hyperreflective material (arrow) but no subretinal fluid. (D) Repeat OCT 1 month later shows new intraretinal edema (arrowhead), subretinal fluid (*), and enlargement of the subretinal hyperreflective material (arrow), consistent with a CNV. (Reprinted with permission from Sundeep K. Kasi, MD.)

- Indocyanine green angiography: early hypercyanescence may reveal disorganized choriocapillaris in cases of CNV
- Optical coherence tomography (OCT): shows location and extent of CNV; useful for monitoring disease activity and response to therapy (Figures 3-6C and 3-6D)
- Fundus autofluorescence: small, non-pigmented chorioretinal scars appear hypoautofluorescent
- Histoplasmin skin antigen testing: not necessary for diagnosis or routinely performed but can help identify prior exposure to *H. capsulatum*

Differential Diagnosis

Multifocal choroiditis with panuveitis, multiple evanescent white dot syndrome (MEWDS), myopic degeneration, punctate inner choroidopathy, sarcoidosis, serpiginous choroiditis, choroidal rupture with choroidal neovascularization, age-related macular degeneration

Management

Monitor for development of CNV; anti-vascular endothelial growth factor injections are the primary treatment for CNV

CANDIDA CHORIORETINITIS

Joshua H. Uhr, MD and
Sunir J. Garg, MD, FACS

- Ocular candidiasis is uncommon, with recent studies reporting rates as low as 1% in those with candidemia. Occurs in patients with candidemia via hematogenous spread to the choroid and retina through capillaries, with potential breakthrough into the vitreous.
- Usually endogenous but can be exogenous (eg, trauma). Risk factors for ocular candidiasis: infection with *Candida albicans* (vs non-albicans Candida species); multiple positive blood cultures; immunosuppression, either due to illness or medications

Signs and Symptoms

May be asymptomatic due to an indolent course; blurred vision, pain, photophobia

Exam Findings

- Chorioretinitis: focal, deep, yellow-white lesions without vitritis (Figure 3-7A)
- Endophthalmitis: vitritis and "fluff balls" in vitreous; may have hypopyon, scleritis, and optic nerve involvement

Testing

OCT has 2 patterns:

- Chorioretinal infiltration: eruption from choroid through the retinal pigment epithelium (RPE) with progression through the retinal layers (Figure 3-7B)
- Retinovascular infiltration without choroidal involvement: fungal "emboli" leading to focal vasculitis, nerve fiber layer infarction

Differential Diagnosis

- Infectious (bacterial endophthalmitis, acute retinal necrosis, toxoplasmosis chorioretinitis, tuberculosis); inflammatory (intermediate/posterior uveitis, sarcoidosis, Behçet's disease, Vogt-Koyanagi-Harada disease); neoplastic (retinoblastoma, intraocular lymphoma, leukemic infiltrate)

Management

- Systemic antifungal therapy: consider in patients with chorioretinitis (no vitritis) that does not involve the macula
  - Oral fluconazole (if susceptible) 800 mg (12 mg/kg) loading dose, then 400 to 800 mg (6 to 12 mg/kg) once a day
  - Intravenous voriconazole 400 mg (6 mg/kg) every 12 hours for 2 doses, then 300 mg (4 mg/kg) every 12 hours

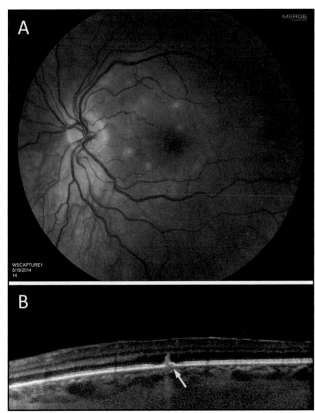

Figure 3-7. (A) Localized deep white chorioretinal lesions, characteristic of Candida chorioretinitis, without vitritis. (B) Enhanced-depth imaging OCT of the same eye shows a focal sub-RPE infiltrate with RPE breakthrough (arrow). (Reprinted with permission from Sonia Mehta, MD.)

- Intravitreal antifungal therapy: use in conjunction with systemic antifungals if macula is threatened or vitritis is present
  - Amphotericin B deoxycholate 5 to 10 µg/0.1 mL or voriconazole 100 µg/0.1 mL
- Surgery (eg, PPV): may be necessary in recalcitrant cases or to obtain specimen for diagnostic testing
- Treatment course is usually 4 to 6 weeks or until all lesions have resolved on serial funduscopic examinations
- In patients with candidemia without ocular involvement, a repeat exam should be performed every 2 weeks

Syphilitic Chorioretinitis

Douglas R. Matsunaga, MD and
Sonia Mehta, MD

- Syphilis is a sexually transmitted infection caused by the spirochete *Treponema pallidum* that may involve almost any structure in the eye.
- Most common ocular presentations: panuveitis and posterior uveitis with chorioretinitis
- Manifestation of secondary syphilis
- May be unilateral or bilateral and may or may not present with systemic symptoms

Signs and Symptoms

Decreased vision, floaters

Exam Findings

One or more placoid, yellow, outer retinal lesions (Figure 3-8A); may have associated anterior uveitis, vitritis, retinal vasculitis, serous/exudative retinal detachment (RD) or papillitis

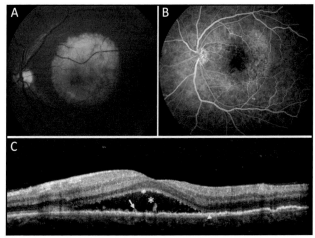

Figure 3-8. (A) Color fundus photograph showing an outer retinal yellow placoid syphilitic lesion. (B) FA in venous phase showing hyperfluorescence of the lesion with scattered hypofluorescent spots. (C) OCT of syphilitic lesion showing areas of retinal pigment epithelial nodularity (arrow), subretinal fluid (*), and scattered punctate hyperreflective spots in the choroid (arrowhead).

Testing

- Labs
  - Non-treponemal tests: rapid plasma reagin (RPR), venereal disease research laboratory (VDRL)
    - High sensitivity semi-quantitative tests that measure antibodies against antigens released by damaged host cells and spirochetes; titers may be used to track active disease, follow treatment response, or reinfection
  - Treponemal tests: fluorescent treponemal antibody absorption (FTA-ABS), *T. pallidum*, enzyme immunoassay (EIA), treponemal pallidum particle agglutination

- Highly specific qualitative tests that measure antibodies against *T pallidum* proteins; remains positive for life
  - The Centers for Disease Control and Prevention recommends obtaining both types of testing for accurate diagnosis via "reverse sequence" testing which starts with a nonspecific immunoassay such as EIA. If negative, syphilis is ruled out. If positive, a non-treponemal test such as RPR is performed with a positive being diagnostic of syphilis. A negative RPR following a positive EIA is a discordant result that must be confirmed by a different treponemal test such as treponemal pallidum particle agglutination which is very sensitive and specific.
  - Screening for the human immunodeficiency virus (HIV) is important due to high rate of co-infection.
- Lumbar puncture (LP): cerebrospinal fluid (CSF) VDRL and analysis
- FA: Early hypofluorescence with increasing hyperfluorescence in mid and late phase images. Scattered hypofluorescent spots ("leopard spotting"; Figure 3-8B)
- OCT: may show hyperreflective RPE nodularity with disorganization of the ellipsoid zone, subretinal fluid, and/or punctate hyperreflectivity in the choroid (Figure 3-8C)

Differential Diagnosis

Viral retinitis (eg, progressive outer retinal necrosis [PORN], acute retinal necrosis [ARN], cytomegalovirus [CMV] retinitis), white dot syndrome (eg, acute posterior multifocal placoid pigment epitheliopathy, multifocal choroiditis), sarcoidosis, tuberculosis, neoplastic (eg, subretinal lymphoma, metastasis)

Management

- Infectious disease consultation is recommended for LP and assist in medical treatment
- Treat as neurosyphilis: penicillin G sodium (18 to 24 million units once a day) or penicillin G procaine (2.4 million units intramuscular once a day) plus probenecid by mouth for 10 to 14 days
- Repeat LP is indicated at 6 months post-treatment if initial CSF VDRL is positive

ACUTE RETINAL NECROSIS

Kalla A. Gervasio, MD and
Sunir J. Garg, MD, FACS

- Caused by infection with varicella zoster virus (VZV; more common in older patients) or herpes simplex virus (HSV; more common in younger patients); less often by CMV or Epstein-Barr virus (EBV)
- Usually presents in fifth to seventh decade of life in immunocompetent adults
- Two-thirds of cases are unilateral, 1/3 are bilateral

Signs and Symptoms

Acute decrease in vision, photophobia, eye pain, redness, flashes, floaters, visual field loss

Exam Findings

- American Uveitis Society criteria: one or more foci of retinitis and/or necrosis with discrete borders in periphery (Figure 3-9), circumferential spread, occlusive vasculopathy with arterial involvement, prominent inflammation in the

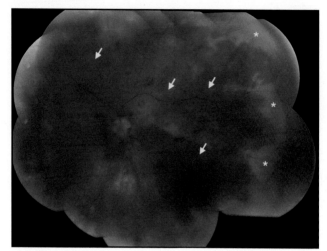

Figure 3-9. Wide-field fundus photograph of a left eye demonstrating multiple foci of retinal necrosis (*) with discrete borders in the periphery, vascular sheathing, occlusive vasculopathy (arrows), and retinal hemorrhages consistent with ARN. Optic disc edema is also evident.

anterior chamber and/or vitreous, rapid disease progression in absence of antiviral medication

- Additional findings: keratic precipitates, conjunctival injection, episcleritis or scleritis, elevated IOP, vascular sheathing, retinal hemorrhages, optic disc edema, delayed onset RD (70% of cases)

Testing

- Labs: HIV, complete blood count, RPR/VDRL, FTA-ABS, erythrocyte sedimentation rate, toxoplasma titers, purified protein derivative (PPD) or QuantiFERON-TB Gold
- Anterior chamber or vitreous paracentesis: viral and toxoplasma PCR

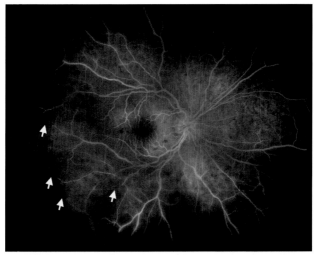

Figure 3-10. FA of a right eye demonstrating retinal vasculitis and ischemia with diffuse leakage of dye from retinal veins and vascular obstruction (arrows) in the peripheral fundus.

- FA: reveals extent of retinal vasculitis and ischemia (Figure 3-10)
- Computed tomography/MRI scan of brain and/or LP: if suspicion for malignancy, syphilis, or encephalitis

Differential Diagnosis

PORN, CMV retinitis, toxoplasma chorioretinitis, syphilis, Behçet's disease, sarcoidosis, fungal or bacterial endophthalmitis, intraocular lymphoma or leukemia

Management

- Medication
  - Oral antiviral and intravitreal injections

- Valacyclovir 1 to 2 g by mouth 3 times a day or famciclovir 500 mg 3 times a day (first-line treatment) or acyclovir 800 mg 5 times a day (second-line treatment)
  - Intravitreal foscarnet or ganciclovir once to twice a week
  ○ Alternative regimen: Intravenous antiviral medications with intravitreal injections followed by oral antiviral
    - Intravenous acyclovir 10 mg/kg 3 times a day for 5 to 14 days
    - Intravitreal foscarnet or ganciclovir once to twice a week
    - Valacyclovir 1 g by mouth 3 times a day or acyclovir 400 to 800 mg 5 times a day
  ○ Duration of either regimen is up to 14 weeks from infection onset
- Treat anterior chamber inflammation with topical steroid and cycloplegic medication
- If optic nerve is involved, consider oral corticosteroids after 24 hours of antiviral therapy (prednisone 60 to 80 mg once a day by mouth for 1 to 2 weeks followed by gradual taper)
- Laser photocoagulation posterior to active retinitis is of unclear efficacy as prophylaxis against rhegmatogenous retinal detachment (RRD)
- PPV with gas or silicone oil for RRD

PROGRESSIVE OUTER RETINAL NECROSIS

Joshua H. Uhr, MD and
James P. Dunn, MD

- Necrotizing herpetic retinopathy usually caused by VZV, often bilateral at presentation or progresses to become bilateral

- Occurs in profoundly immunosuppressed patients (CD4 + lymphocyte usually < 50 cells/μL), predominantly with advanced HIV

Signs and Symptoms

Rapid onset of painless decreased vision, visual field constriction, floaters

Exam Findings

Often concurrent cutaneous zoster (may be in dermatomes remote from eye or may be temporally remote from onset of PORN); multiple areas of discrete yellow-white opacities of outer retina, which rapidly coalesce, in periphery or macula (up to 1/3 of cases present with macular lesions); may have perivascular sparing of confluent lesions; minimal or no intraocular inflammation or vasculitis; hemorrhages uncommon; retinal breaks in necrotic areas often lead to RD; retinal atrophy, attenuated vessels, and pigment mottling following resolution (Figure 3-11)

Testing

- Identification of causative virus by PCR of intraocular fluid may be useful for guiding antiviral therapy; check for VZV, HSV-1 and 2, CMV
- HIV testing, if not previously diagnosed

Differential Diagnosis

ARN (Table 3-1), CMV retinitis, endophthalmitis (fungal or bacterial), syphilitic retinitis, sarcoidosis, tuberculosis, toxoplasmosis, lymphoma, metastatic disease

Management

- Given rarity of this disease, optimal treatment regimen is unclear, but combination of intravenous and intravitreal

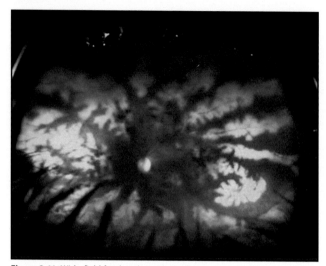

Figure 3-11. Wide-field fundus photograph of an eye with PORN demonstrating coalescing areas of retinal opacification in the posterior pole and periphery, some hemorrhages in the necrotic regions, and a notable absence of significant vitritis. (Reprinted with permission from Bryn M. Burkholder, MD.)

Table 3-1. Features Distinguishing Progressive Outer Retinal Necrosis from Acute Retinal Necrosis

	PORN	ARN
Etiology	Usually VZV	VZV, HSV-1 (older patients), HSV-2 (younger patients)
Lesion Location	Peripheral or macular	Peripheral, beyond arcades
Patient Immune Status	Compromised	Competent or compromised
Presence of Intraocular Inflammation	No (if present, minimal)	Yes (vitritis and anterior chamber cell)
Presence of Pain	No	Often painful
Status of Retinal Vessels	Perivascular sparing	Occlusive vasculitis

therapy appears to have better outcomes than intravenous antivirals alone

- Various combinations of systemic and intravitreal antivirals have been reported
  - ○ Systemic antiviral options: vidarabine, famciclovir, cidofovir, foscarnet, ganciclovir, or acyclovir
  - ○ Intravitreal antiviral options: ganciclovir (2 mg/0.05 mL) and foscarnet (1.2 mg/0.05 mL)
- Highly active antiretroviral therapy (HAART) therapy likely reduces progression
- Laser barricade of necrotic retina to lower risk of RD is of unproven benefit due to rapid progression of retinitis
- Repair of RD usually requires silicone oil tamponade
- Retinitis may recur (usually with a decreased dose, switch, or cessation of antivirals), in contrast to ARN

CYTOMEGALOVIRUS RETINITIS

Christopher M. Aderman, MD

- CMV is a double-stranded DNA herpesvirus most commonly seen as an opportunistic infection in acquired immunodeficiency syndrome (AIDS) but may arise from other causes of systemic immunosuppression. Risk of CMV retinitis increases with CD4 count < 50 cells/mm^3.
- Prior to HAART, CMV retinitis affected 30% of AIDS patients. With the advent of HAART, the incidence of CMV retinitis has decreased dramatically to 0.36 cases per 100 person-years in AIDS patients.
- CMV spreads hematogenously to infect the retinovascular endothelium, resulting in a full-thickness retinal infection that can lead to severe vision loss, RD, and blindness.

Signs and Symptoms

Painless vision loss, flashes, floaters, blind spots; may be asymptomatic depending on the location and extent of retinal involvement, or due to an inability to mount an immune response

Exam Findings

- While very early CMV may resemble extra-large cotton wool spots, most early CMV lesions arise as small foci of hemorrhagic retinitis in a perivascular distribution. Less often, it may originate at the optic nerve or retinal periphery.
- Three patterns of retinitis
  - Fulminant: yellow-white lesions with hemorrhagic necrosis often centered around the vasculature in a wedge shape distribution (Figures 3-12 and 3-13)
  - Granular: seen more often in the retinal periphery with little to no necrosis and hemorrhage
  - Perivascular: diffuse perivascular exudate and retinal whitening with the appearance of a "frosted branch angiitis"
- Three zones of involvement
  - Zone 1: (imminently sight threatening) 1 disc diameter around the disc and 2 disc diameters around the fovea
  - Zone 2: anterior to Zone 1, posterior to vortex veins
  - Zone 3: peripheral to Zone 2

Testing

- Fundus photography can be used to document lesion progression. FA is usually not necessary, but will show vascular non-perfusion and blockage from retinal hemorrhages.
- Diagnostic tests for CMV viremia, blood antigen, or blood culture are not helpful due to poor sensitivity and specificity for determining CMV end-organ disease

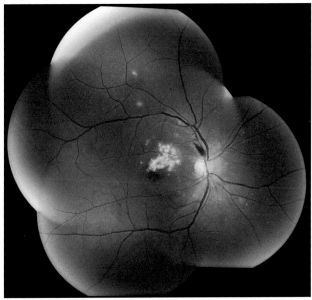

Figure 3-12. Fundus photograph of CMV retinitis in 56-year-old man with AIDS (CD4 + 10 cells/mm³) on HAART therapy but with HIV antiretroviral resistance.

- PCR analysis of aqueous or vitreous fluid can be done in cases where diagnosis uncertain

Differential Diagnosis

HIV retinopathy, ARN, PORN, toxoplasmosis, histoplasmosis, syphilis, lymphoma

Management

- Prevention: for those with HIV/AIDS, HAART and regular follow-up with an infectious disease specialist is critical
- Screening: patients with CD4 count < 50 cells/mm³ should be examined at least every 3 months

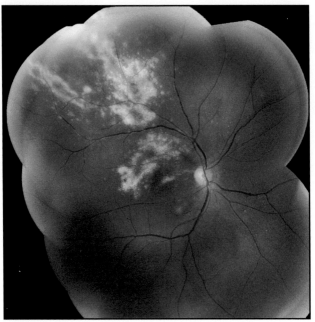

Figure 3-13. CMV retinitis continued to worsen despite valganciclovir, concerning for valganciclovir resistance. Unfortunately, the patient was unable to switch to intravenous foscarnet due to poor liver function in the setting of plasmablastic lymphoma. Fundus photograph shows progression of retinitis.

- Systemic
  - Oral valganciclovir (preferred treatment)—induction: 900 mg twice a day for 2 to 3 weeks; maintenance: 900 mg once a day
  - Intravenous ganciclovir—induction: 5 mg/kg twice a day for 2 weeks; maintenance: 5 mg/kg once a day

- ○ Intravenous foscarnet—induction: 60 mg/kg every 8 hours for 2 weeks; maintenance: 90 mg/kg once a day
  - ○ Intravenous cidofovir—induction: 5 mg/kg once a week for 2 weeks; maintenance: 3 mg/kg every 2 weeks
- Intravitreal (to be used in conjunction with systemic therapy in patients with imminently sight-threatening lesions)
  - ○ Intravitreal ganciclovir—induction: 2 mg twice a week for 3 weeks; maintenance: 2 mg once a week
  - ○ Ganciclovir implant (no longer commercially available)—induction: 4.5 mg implant; maintenance: replace every 6 to 8 months
  - ○ Intravitreal foscarnet—induction: 2.4 mg twice a week for 3 weeks; maintenance: 2.4 mg once a week
  - ○ Intravitreal cidofovir—induction: 20 μg; maintenance: repeat every 5 to 6 weeks
  - ○ Intravitreal fomivirsen—induction: 300 μg every 2 weeks for 4 weeks; maintenance: 300 μg every 4 weeks
- Endpoint for maintenance therapy is when the following conditions are met:
  - ○ Retinitis is quiescent with no lesion progression
  - ○ Retinitis has been treated with anti-CMV therapy for 3 months
  - ○ HIV viral load is suppressed and CD4 count increases to ≥ 100 for at least 3 months
- Following treatment, CMV retinitis that is no longer active appears as atrophic retinal lesions. Reactivation usually occurs at the edge of past lesions.
- Secondary complications include the following:
  - ○ Immune recovery uveitis—as CD4 counts increase with HAART, anterior and/or intermediate uveitis can arise as the immune system responds to CMV antigens
  - ○ Rhegmatogenous RD—more common if involvement exceeds 25% of the retina

HUMAN IMMUNODEFICIENCY VIRUS RETINOPATHY

Philip P. Storey, MD, MPH and
James P. Dunn, MD

- Most common ocular manifestation of HIV
- Potential causes: immune complex deposition, direct invasion of virus into vascular endothelium, or increased plasma viscosity
- Incidence strongly correlated with degree of HIV disease with incidence > 50% when CD4+ count <100 cells/mL

Signs and Symptoms

Usually asymptomatic; visual fields may show small scotomata; with progressive disease, subtle optic neuropathy with decreased color vision and contrast sensitivity may occur; narrowed retinal arterioles may be a marker of progressive neurologic disease and premature aging

Exam Findings

Cotton wool spots (Figure 3-14A): opacification resolves as edema clears; retinal hemorrhages: dot/blot and/or flame shaped; microvascular changes: microaneurysms, telangiectasia; severe retinitis or choroiditis in the setting of HIV likely indicates an opportunistic infection due to disseminated disease

Testing

- Usually none required
- FA: may show microvascular abnormalities and non-perfusion (Figure 3-14B)
- CD4+ T-cell count, HIV viral load: determine disease severity and level of immunosuppression

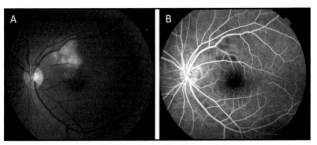

Figure 3-14. HIV retinopathy. (A) Color fundus photo with large cotton wool spot. (B) FA showing corresponding capillary non-perfusion and vascular staining. (Reprinted with permission from David C. Reed, MD.)

Differential Diagnosis

CMV retinitis, hypertensive retinopathy, diabetic retinopathy, necrotizing herpetic retinitis, syphilitic retinitis, metastatic fungal endophthalmitis, leukemic retinopathy, pancreatitis, Purtscher's retinopathy, drug-induced retinopathy (eg, interferon)

Management

- Immune recovery with combination antiretroviral therapy (HAART)
- Management of other vasculopathic risk factors (eg, cigarette smoking, hypertension, diabetes, hyperlipidemia)
- Treatment of underlying infections or malignancy

OCULAR TOXOCARIASIS

Daniel Su, MD and
Maxwell S. Stem, MD

- Intraocular infection most commonly caused by a parasitic nematode of the *Ascaridia* family called *Toxocara canis* (or less commonly *Toxocara cati*), a natural parasite of puppies (definitive host), rabbits, and rodents

- Humans become infected via ingestion of eggs or larvae found in soil, contaminated hands and/or undercooked meats and from the small intestine are disseminated to viscera and eye via hematogenous spread
- Estimated to account for approximately 1% of all cases of uveitis among all age groups referred to tertiary care centers in the United States
- Systemic *Toxocara canis* infections often involve a self-limiting constellation of features referred to as visceral larva migrans (VLM): fever, pallor, anorexia, malaise, wheeze, cough, and moderate eosinophilia. However, more serious complications have been reported (pneumonia, congestive heart failure, and convulsions).

Signs and Symptoms

Usually unilateral decreased vision, pain, photophobia, floaters, leukocoria, strabismus

Exam Findings

Anterior chamber cell (73%), vitritis (100%), retinal granuloma is a common ocular finding located in the peripheral retina approximately 50% of the time, often fibrocellular bands extend from the peripheral granuloma to the posterior pole (posterior retina or optic disc) resulting in tractional retinal folds which can cause RD and/or macular dragging (Figure 3-15)

Testing

- B-scan ultrasound may reveal granuloma
- Histologic demonstration of larva is the definitive diagnosis, but this is rarely performed
- Serologic testing for anti-*Toxocara canis* antibodies in serum or aqueous via enzyme-linked immunosorbent assay (ELISA) is a valuable test with relatively high sensitivity

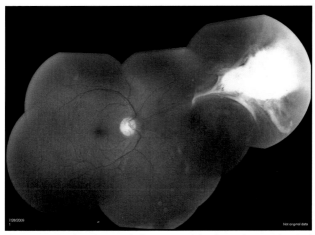

Figure 3-15. Fundus photograph depicts a peripheral granuloma with retinal traction. The macula is not involved.

- Cytologic testing (ie, identification of eosinophils) may be helpful in identifying intraocular toxocariasis infection
- OCT of posterior pole granulomas usually demonstrates a highly-reflective mass located above RPE
- Note: evaluation of stool for ova and parasites is not necessary as humans do not shed parasite

Differential Diagnosis

Retinoblastoma, retinopathy of prematurity, Coats disease, persistent fetal vasculature syndrome, familiar exudative vitreoretinopathy, toxoplasmosis, tuberculosis, syphilis, sarcoidosis

Management

- Quiescent disease without active infection can be observed
- If active inflammation is present
  - Topical cycloplegic and topical and/or systemic steroids

- ○ Antihelminth therapy: its role is controversial but when used in combination with steroids, good results have been reported

- ○ Oral albendazole is most commonly used (800 mg twice a day for adults and 400 mg twice a day for children), typically for 1 month

- ○ If a subretinal larva is visible, laser can be used to destroy it

- ○ In rare instance where choroidal neovascularization occurs, management with intravitreal anti-VEGF therapy can be considered

- Surgical intervention is needed in cases of vitreous opacification, RD, cataract or glaucoma

DIFFUSE UNILATERAL SUBACUTE NEURORETINOPATHY

Nikolas J. S. London, MD

- Etiology: nematode invasion of the subretinal space by *Baylisascaris procyonis*, *Ancylostoma caninum*, *Toxocara canis*, or *Dirofilaria*

- Likely fecal-oral or fecal-cutaneous infection

- Most commonly unilateral and more common in children and young adults

- Early and late stages: starts as deep gray-white lesions and optic nerve head edema; advanced cases develop optic atrophy, vascular attenuation, and visual field loss

Signs and Symptoms

No systemic symptoms; patients may have no ocular symptoms; central or paracentral scotoma, mild visual acuity decline, positive afferent pupillary defect (APD)

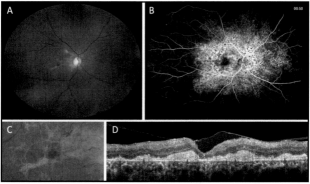

Figure 3-16. Diffuse unilateral subacute neuroretinitis. (A) Wide-field fundus photo demonstrating near confluent retinal pigment epithelial clumping and macular subretinal fibrosis. (B) Wide-field FA shows widespread hyperfluorescence with punctate hypofluorescence corresponding to the pigment clumping. (C) Close-up view of the macula reveals the subretinal nematode (arrow). (D) OCT demonstrates diffuse RPE atrophy and outer retinal disorganization with hyperreflective clumps (arrowheads) corresponding to subretinal fibrosis. (Reprinted with permission from J. Michael Jumper, MD.)

Exam Findings

- Early: Scattered deep retinal, gray-white retinal lesions, < 1 disc diameter each with mild-moderate vitritis, optic nerve head edema, and hyperemia. Nematode may be visible with careful contact-lens biomicroscopy (Figure 3-16C). Lesion typically resolve over days to weeks.
- Late: diffuse RPE atrophy with optic atrophy (Figure 3-16A), vascular attenuation, vitritis, visual loss, and a prominent APD

Testing

- FA: Early hypofluorescence and late leakage from areas of retinitis. Leakage from optic nerve edema and vasculitis, if present (Figure 3-16B).

- OCT: loss of RPE layer and outer retinal bands; subretinal fibrosis manifesting as hyperreflective subretinal material in advanced cases (Figure 3-16D)
- Scanning laser ophthalmoscopy with blue illumination may assist in localizing the nematode (appears white on a dark background)
- Visual field exam may show paracentral or central scotomas
- Laboratory workup is of minimal value and not typically performed

Differential Diagnosis

Ocular toxoplasmosis, herpetic retinitis, acute posterior multifocal placoid pigment epitheliopathy (APMPPE), ocular histoplasmosis, sardoidosis, syphilis, MEWDS

Management

- If nematode is visible on exam it can be destroyed with retinal laser
- Oral antihelminithics are controversial, but may be the only option in cases where the nematode is not readily visible. Options include: albendazole 200 mg twice a day for 30 days; ivermectin 0.15 to 0.20 mg/kg once a day and thiabendazole 25 mg/kg once a day in 2 divided doses for 2 to 4 days

EALES DISEASE

Sasha Hubschman, MD and
Jayanth Sridhar, MD

- Vascular inflammation in peripheral retina with predilection for veins
- Usually occurs in 20 to 30 year old males (especially from Indian subcontinent)

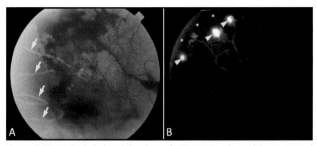

Figure 3-17. (A) Occluded peripheral venules (arrows) with overlying preretinal hemorrhage in Eales disease with FA confirming non-perfusion (*) and (B) leakage (arrowheads). (Reprinted with permission from Audina M. Berrocal, MD.)

- Typically bilateral but asymmetric as fellow eye may be affected 3 to 10 years later
- A diagnosis of exclusion with unclear etiology, possibly associated with mycobacterium tuberculosis (TB)

Signs and Symptoms

Early disease may be asymptomatic due to peripheral location; advanced disease may have floaters, photopsia, mild to profound painless visual loss caused by vitreous hemorrhage (VH)

Exam Findings

Inflammation (peripheral perivasculitis): can affect all quadrants with venous sheathing as active vasculitis resolves (Figures 3-17A, 3-18A, 3-18B, and 3-18C); occlusion: ischemic changes due to non-perfusion; peripheral retinal neovascularization: sea fan appearance that often leads to recurrent VH (hallmark of disease) and possible tractional retinal detachment (TRD)

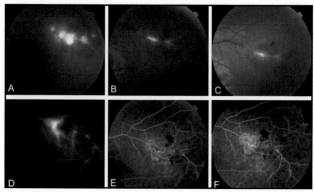

Figure 3-18. Active Eales disease (A, D) with improvement of inflammation and hemorrhage after 1 month of systemic corticosteroids (B, E) and resolution after 3 months total treatment with slow taper (C, F). (Reprinted with permission from John D. Pitcher III, MD.)

Testing

- Labs: complete blood count, urinalysis, erythrocyte sedimentation rate, tuberculin skin test; other tests for retinal vasculitis (antiphospholipid antibodies, rheumatoid factor, anti-cyclic citrullinated peptide antibodies, antineutrophil cytoplasmic antibodies), RPR/VDRL, FTA-ABS, HIV
- Imaging
  - Chest x-ray: exclude sarcoidosis, TB, systemic vasculitis
  - FA: evaluate for non-perfusion, neovascularization (Figures 3-17B, 3-18D, 3-18E, and 3-18F)
  - B-scan ultrasound: if VH is present to evaluate for TRD

Differential Diagnosis

Branch retinal vein occlusion, proliferative diabetic retinopathy, diseases with peripheral retinal non-perfusion (Coats disease, familial exudative vitreoretinopathy [FEVR], sickle cell disease); masqueraders: tuberculosis, syphilis, sarcoidosis, necrotizing retinitis (arteries are more commonly involved); idiopathic retinal vasculitis

Management

- Observation if only venous sheathing is seen on exam and follow-up every 6 months with exam and FA
- Sub-Tenon or intravitreal corticosteroid injections (for unilateral disease) if cystoid macular edema is present
- Systemic corticosteroids (for bilateral and severe disease): oral prednisone 1 mg/kg once a day for 1 month with slow taper thereafter (Figure 3-18)
- Methotrexate is a common steroid-sparing treatment option
- Laser photocoagulation: indicated for secondary neovascularization but contraindicated during periods of active inflammation
- Anti-VEGF injections: case reports with bevacizumab suggest some efficacy
- Vitrectomy: if either VH is obscuring central vision or TRD

REFERENCE

1. Endophthalmitis Vitrectomy Study Group. Results of the Endophthalmitis Vitrectomy Study. A randomized trial of immediate vitrectomy and of intravenous antibiotics for the treatment of postoperative bacterial endophthalmitis. *Arch Ophthalmol.* 1995;113(12):1479-1496. doi:10.1001/archopht.1995.01100120009001

4

Noninfectious Inflammatory Diseases

Multifocal Choroiditis

Rebecca R. Soares, MD, MPH and
Sonia Mehta, MD

- Characterized by multifocal chorioretinal inflammatory lesions that leave pigmented fibrotic scars; typically bilateral and not associated with any systemic disease
- Usually occurs in young (~30 years old) Caucasian females with myopia
- Course is typically chronic with recurrent inflammation
- Visual acuity preserved in majority of patients (~65% to 75% retain ≥ 20/40 or better)
- Most common cause of decreased vision is choroidal neovascularization (CNV). Other causes include macular edema, foveal scarring, and epiretinal membrane (ERM).

Hsu J, Chiang A, eds. *The Pocket Guide to Medical Retina* (pp 119-151).
© 2021 Taylor & Francis Group.

Signs and Symptoms

Floaters, blurry vision, scotoma, metamorphopsia, photopsia, photophobia

Exam Findings

Bilateral yellow-white punched out chorioretinal lesions (size 50 to 200 μm) with variable pigmented fibrotic scars in posterior pole and periphery often clustered nasal to disc (Figures 4-1A, 4-1B, and 4-2A); Schlaegel lines: peripheral curvilinear streaks of chorioretinitis; vitritis and anterior chamber inflammation in multifocal choroiditis with panuveitis (MFCPU); other findings: peripapillary atrophy, disc edema, macular edema, retinal detachment, CNV, ERM

Testing

- No diagnostic laboratory test for multifocal choroiditis. Testing may be done to rule out infectious or noninfectious causes. Tuberculosis: QuantiFERON-TB Gold or purified protein derivative; syphilis: rapid plasma reagin (RPR) and fluorescent treponemal antibody absorption (FTA-ABS); sarcoidosis: chest x-ray and angiotensin converting enzyme (ACE); histoplasmosis: urine anion gap and/or serum Ab.

- Fluorescein angiography (FA): early hypofluorescence of lesions followed by late staining; early hyperfluorescence with late leakage if CNV present (Figures 4-1C and 4-1D)

- Indocyanine green (ICG) angiography (ICGA): early and late hypocyanescence of lesions

- Fundus autofluorescence: active lesions—hyperautofluorescence of retinal pigment epithelial (RPE) elevations, central absent autofluorescence if dehiscence of RPE; inactive lesions—absent autofluorescence in areas of RPE scarring or atrophy (Figure 4-2B)

- Optical coherence tomography (OCT): active lesions—RPE elevation with sub-RPE infiltration of homogenous debris

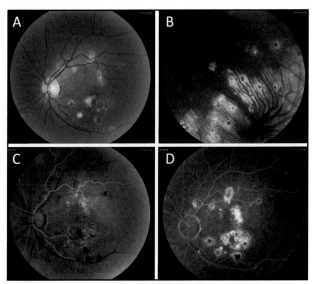

Figure 4-1. Fundus photos of a patient with multifocal choroiditis demonstrating multiple yellow-white punched out chorioretinal lesions some with pigmented scarring in the (A) posterior pole and (B) periphery. FA demonstrating (C) early hypofluorescence followed by (D) hyperfluorescent staining.

and outer retinal changes; CNV—heterogenous subretinal/sub-RPE material, subretinal fluid, intraretinal edema; CME—presence is one indicator of active disease; enhanced depth imaging—increased choroidal thickening in areas corresponding to RPE elevation (Figure 4-2C)

Differential Diagnosis

Presumed ocular histoplasmosis (POHS), punctate inner choroidopathy (PIC), multiple evanescent white dot syndrome (MEWDS), birdshot chorioretinopathy, acute posterior multifocal placoid pigment epitheliopathy (APMPPE), sarcoidosis, tuberculosis (TB), syphilis, toxoplasmosis, candidiasis, lymphoma

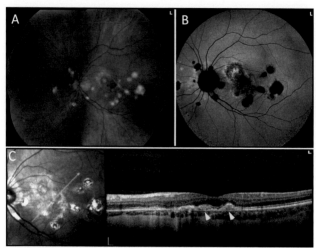

Figure 4-2. (A) Color fundus photo with corresponding (B) fundus autofluorescence revealing hyperautofluorescence of RPE elevations, central absent autofluorescence in areas of RPE dehiscence in active lesions, and absent autofluorescence in areas of RPE scarring or atrophy in inactive lesions. (C) OCT of active lesions showing RPE elevation with sub-RPE infiltration of homogenous debris (arrowheads) and outer retinal changes.

Management

- Treatment favored in the setting of perifoveal active inflammation, macular edema, or CNV
- Periocular or systemic steroids are often first-line treatments for active inflammation
- Immunosuppressive therapy indicated in severe or chronic recurrent cases and reduces risk of posterior pole complications (cystoid macular edema, ERM, and CNV) by 83%
- Intravitreal anti-vascular endothelial growth factor (VEGF) or steroid injections for macular edema and/or CNV

POSTERIOR SCLERITIS

Matthew Trese, DO, MA and
Thomas J. Wubben, MD, PhD

- Rarest form of scleritis and is likely under recognized given significant variability in its clinical presentation. Underlying etiology often idiopathic but there are strong associations with autoimmune and infectious conditions in approximately half of cases.
- Female predominance, primarily unilateral, and may be associated with anterior scleritis

Signs and Symptoms

Periocular pain, blurred vision, headache, photophobia

Exam Findings

Anterior segment may appear normal (unless there is concomitant anterior scleritis), proptosis, or angle closure glaucoma secondary to uveal effusion; posterior segment may have retinal and/or choroidal folds, serous retinal detachment, macular edema, optic disc edema, and subretinal mass due to nodular posterior scleritis

Testing

- Laboratory evaluation is to rule out associated autoimmune and infectious conditions: complete blood count (CBC), rheumatoid factor, anti-CCP, anti-nuclear antibody, antineutrophil cytoplasmic antibodies, ACE, lysozyme, RPR/FTA, QuantiFERON-TB Gold
- Imaging studies may include the following:
  - B-scan ultrasound: posterior scleral thickening (> 2 mm is abnormal) and/or a "T-sign" showing fluid in sub-Tenon's space (Figure 4-3)

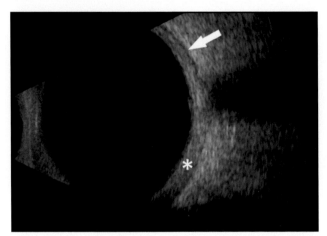

Figure 4-3. B-scan ultrasound demonstrates thickened sclera (*) and fluid in the sub-Tenon's space (arrow, "T-sign").

- Computed tomography or magnetic resonance imaging with contrast: enhancement and thickening of posterior sclera, classically described as a "ring sign" on coronal sections through globe

Differential Diagnosis

Orbital inflammatory syndrome (OIS), idiopathic uveal effusion syndrome, peribulbar mass, central serous retinopathy, uveal lymphoma

Management

- Posterior scleritis poses a significant threat to vision and often mandates more aggressive therapy than anterior scleritis.
- If a systemic disease can be identified, targeted therapy against the infectious or inflammatory process is warranted.

- First-line treatment: oral nonsteroidal anti-inflammatory drugs are generally insufficient; prednisone (1 mg/kg once a day or 60 mg once a day) with gradual tapering depending on clinical response is often required
- Second-line treatment: immunomodulatory therapy such as antimetabolites, alkylating agents or T-cell inhibitors, administered in conjunction with a rheumatologist
- Third-line treatment: biologic agents targeted against tumor necrosis factor alpha (TNF-α) and cluster of differentiation-20 (CD-20) have been used if refractory to systemic steroids and conventional immunomodulatory therapy

MULTIPLE EVANESCENT WHITE DOT SYNDROME

Paul S. Baker, MD

- Acute, unilateral, inflammatory disease characterized by multiple small, white dots in deep retina and retinal pigment epithelium (Figure 4-4A)
- Etiology is unknown, but viral origin and genetic predisposition have been suggested
- Strong female predominance (~75%) and usually affects young adults

Signs and Symptoms

Mild to moderate acute vision loss, usually unilateral; central or temporal scotoma, photopsias; may be preceded by a recent viral flu-like illness

Exam Findings

White dots are concentrated in paramacular area, sparing fovea, which usually has granular appearance with yellowish-orange specks (peau d'orange); vitreous cells, retinal venous sheathing; optic disc edema

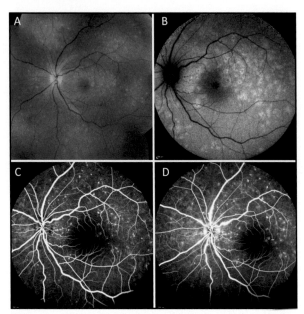

Figure 4-4. MEWDS. (A) Color fundus photo with multiple small white spots. (B) Fundus autofluorescence shows multiple circular areas of hyperautofluorescence that are more widespread and numerous than visible on clinical exam. FA showing (C) early wreath-like hyperfluorescence with (D) late staining. Note the disc hyperfluorescence and leakage along the peripapillary vessels. (Reprinted with permission from Elaine Gonzales.)

Testing

- MEWDS is a clinical diagnosis; there is no diagnostic laboratory testing.
- Fundus autofluorescence: lesions show characteristic hyperautofluorescence which may be more numerous than clinically apparent (Figure 4-4B)
- FA: Early hyperfluorescent spots in a wreath-like configuration with late staining. Optic disc and vascular leakage is often present (Figures 4-4C and 4-4D).

- ICG: more numerous hypocyanescent lesions than expected based on clinical exam; peripapillary hypocyanescence
- OCT: subtle disruption of photoreceptor layer
- Electroretinogram (ERG): reduced a-wave and early receptor potential (ERP) amplitudes
- Visual field testing: enlarged blind spot

Differential Diagnosis

Acute idiopathic blind spot enlargement (AIBSE), acute macular neuroretinopathy (AMN), acute multifocal posterior pigment epitheliopathy (AMPPE), acute retinal pigment epitheliitis, MFCP, PIC, acute zonal occult outer retinopathy (AZOOR), birdshot retinochoroidopathy, primary intraocular lymphoma

Management

Observation as usually self-limited over 1 to 2 months with excellent vision recovery

ACUTE POSTERIOR MULTIFOCAL PLACOID PIGMENT EPITHELIOPATHY

David Xu, MD and
Sonia Mehta, MD

- Rare, idiopathic, bilateral inflammatory condition that usually affects young patients 20 to 40 years old with equal sex predilection
- One-third experience a flu-like prodrome
- Uncommonly associated with central nervous system (CNS) vasculitis or meningoencephalitis

Signs and Symptoms

Acute onset blurry vision, metamorphopsia, and scotomas with bilateral or sequential onset; antecedent flu-like syndrome or upper respiratory illness; headache, hearing loss, stroke, and other neurologic symptoms

Exam Findings

- Acute: mild vitritis; multifocal creamy yellow-white placoid retinal lesions in the posterior pole to mid-periphery at the level of the RPE and choroid (Figure 4-5)
- Chronic: lesions usually fade over 1 to 2 weeks and new lesions may develop; may leave patches of variably pigmented RPE atrophy

Testing

- FA: early hypofluorescence of lesions followed by late staining (Figures 4-6A and 4-6B)
- ICG angiography: early and late hypocyanescence of lesions; more lesions are seen on ICG than clinically apparent (see Figures 4-6A and 4-6B)
- Fundus autofluorescence: hyperautofluorescence of lesions
- OCT: lesions show hyperreflectivity from ellipsoid zone to outer plexiform layer (Figure 4-7)
- OCT angiography: areas of flow deficit in the choriocapillaris corresponding to the placoid lesions

Differential Diagnosis

MEWDS, serpiginous choroidopathy, relentless placoid choroiditis, multifocal choroiditis, Vogt-Koyanagi-Harada syndrome, syphilitic chorioretinitis, tuberculosis, fungal disease, choroidal metastasis, lymphoma

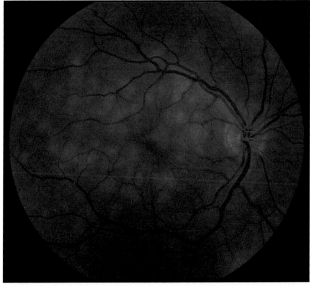

Figure 4-5. Fundus photo of a right eye with acute APMPPE demonstrating bilateral creamy-yellow placoid lesions.

Management

- Generally self-limited and can be observed for resolution
- If patients have neurologic symptoms, workup for CNS involvement with brain MRI and magnetic resonance angiography or CT angiography
- CNS vasculitis should be treated with high-dose IV corticosteroid therapy.
  - Long-term immunosuppression with azathioprine, cyclophosphamide or other steroid-sparing immunomodulators can be considered.

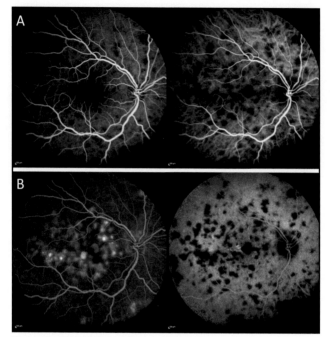

Figure 4-6. (A) Simultaneous fluorescein (left) and ICGA (right) in the early phase demonstrating hypofluorescence and hypocyanescence. (B) Simultaneous fluorescein and ICGA in the late phase demonstrating staining on FA (left) and persistent hypocyanescence (right) on ICG.

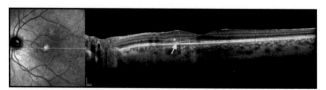

Figure 4-7. OCT of the left eye of a different patient with disruption of the ellipsoid zone (arrow) and hyperreflectivity of the outer nuclear layer (*).

Serpiginous Chorioretinitis

Alok S. Bansal, MD

- Rare, bilateral, asymmetric form of posterior uveitis with characteristic pattern of lesions creeping away from optic disc; recurrences are common
- More common in males; typically affects patients 30 to 70 years old

Signs and Symptoms

Painless vision loss with central or paracentral scotoma, metamorphopsia

Exam Findings

Subretinal yellow-gray patches at level of RPE that typically spread centrifugally from peripapillary area (Figure 4-8A); leading edge of creamy infiltrates with possible subretinal fluid; resolved lesions show chorioretinal atrophy; CNV may develop at edge of an old scar; minimal anterior chamber reaction and/or vitritis

Additional Subtypes

- Macular serpiginous: initial macular lesion sparing peripapillary region with high-risk of CNV
- Ampiginous (relentless placoid): multifocal plaque-like lesions similar to APMPPE but without spontaneous resolution

Testing

- FA: blockage in early phase and staining of leading edge in late phase

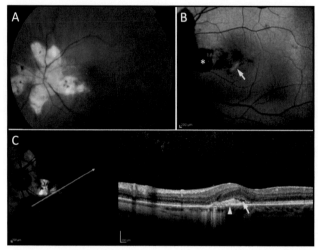

Figure 4-8. Serpiginous chorioretinopathy. (A) Color fundus photo showing pseudopodal appearance of chorioretinal atrophy radiating from optic disc. (B) Fundus autofluorescence showing an area of activity with hyperautofluorescence (arrow) and older, inactive hypoautofluorescent areas (*). (C) OCT demonstrates subretinal fluid (yellow arrow) adjacent to an active hyperreflective subretinal lesion (arrowhead).

- Fundus autofluorescence: hypoautofluorescence of inactive areas and hyperautofluorescence of active disease areas (Figure 4-8B)
- OCT: may show subretinal fluid or loss of RPE (Figure 4-8C)
- Labs: tuberculin skin testing or QuantiFERON-TB Gold

Differential Diagnosis

APMPPE, multifocal choroiditis, toxoplasmosis, serpiginous-like choroidopathy related to tuberculosis infection, other white dot syndromes or causes of posterior uveitis (sarcoid, syphilis)

Management

Immunosuppression with combination corticosteroids (systemic, periocular, and/or intravitreal) and steroid-sparing agents such as methotrexate, cyclosporine A, or azathioprine. Given high incidence of recurrence, some patients may require chronic therapy.

BIRDSHOT CHORIORETINOPATHY

Connie M. Wu, MD and
James P. Dunn, MD

- Autoimmune retinopathy of unknown cause although strong HLA-A29 gene correlation
- Most common white dot syndrome (0.5% to 1.5% of all uveitis)
- Older adults, 30 to 70 years old; females > males; more common in Caucasians
- Bilateral, may be asymmetric; insidious onset with chronic course; recurrences are common

Signs and Symptoms

Floaters, peripheral photopsias, decreased night vision and color vision, visual field constriction; vision may be affected by macular edema, macular atrophy, optic disc atrophy, or CNV

Exam Findings

Usually mild anterior uveitis, mild to moderate intermediate uveitis; vitritis with ovoid yellowish, off-white posterior retinal lesions 50 to 1500 μm, distributed radially from optic nerve, often along underlying choroidal vasculature; lesions do not become pigmented over time (Figure 4-9)

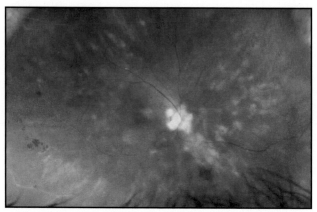

Figure 4-9. Wide-field fundus image of right eye with classic late birdshot chorioretinopathy, including vitritis with ovoid yellowish, off-white posterior retinal lesions 50 to 1500 µm, distributed radially from optic nerve, along underlying choroidal vasculature.

- Acute findings: vasculitis, cystoid macular edema, optic disc inflammation
- Late findings: disc atrophy, ERM, CNV

Testing

- Positive HLA-A29 test in > 96% of cases (high negative predictive value, but limited positive predictive value unless exam findings are consistent with birdshot chorioretinopathy)
- FA: variable; may show retinal vasculitis, macular leakage, and vascular staining (Figure 4-10)
- ICGA: better demonstrates hypocyanescence corresponding to choroidal infiltrates
- OCT: macular edema, disruption of ellipsoid zone, suprachoroidal fluid, foveal thinning, progressive choroidal thinning despite clinically inactive disease

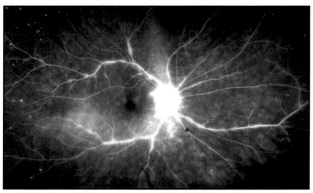

Figure 4-10. Wide-field fluorescein angiogram of right eye reveals disc hyperfluorescence, vasculitis with vascular staining, and punctate peripheral leakage.

- OCT angiography: may show hypoperfusion corresponding to ICGA abnormalities
- Fundus autofluorescence: hyperautofluorescent lesions in regions of RPE atrophy not necessarily matching clinically apparent lesions with possible placoid macular hypoautofluorescence
- Goldmann visual field better than automated 30-2 Humphrey visual fields at showing diffuse peripheral constriction
- Electroretinography: not commonly used, but may show diminished b-wave in active disease and improvement with immunosuppressive therapy

Differential Diagnosis

Multifocal choroiditis, lymphoma, APMPPE

Management

- A small percentage of patients may not progress and can be monitored, however a majority require chronic immunosuppression with corticosteroids (regional or sustained-release implants) or immunomodulatory therapy

- Immunosuppressive therapy (early addition advised given that a majority fail to resolve on steroids alone)
  - Antimetabolites (eg, azathioprine, methotrexate, mycophenolate mofetil)
  - Calcineurin inhibitors (eg, tacrolimus, cyclosporine)
  - TNF antagonists (eg, adalimumab, infliximab)
- For macular edema:
  - Intravitreal preferable to periocular corticosteroid injections
  - Intravitreal anti-VEGF injections (eg, aflibercept, bevacizumab, ranibizumab)

OCULAR SARCOIDOSIS

Adam T. Gerstenblith, MD

- Multisystem granulomatous disorder of unknown etiology
- Pulmonary involvement is most common; ocular involvement occurs in approximately 15% to 50% of patients with systemic sarcoidosis; 10 to 20 times more prevalent in African-Americans than Caucasians in the United States

Signs and Symptoms

Blurring of vision, aching or pain in and around the eyes, photophobia, floaters

Exam Findings

Acute or chronic granulomatous anterior uveitis is most common presentation: mutton-fat keratic precipitates; Koeppe (pupillary border) and Busacca (mid-peripheral) iris nodules; advanced

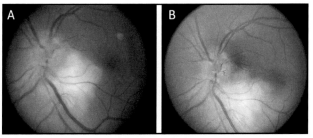

Figure 4-11. (A) Color fundus photo of choroidal and optic disc granuloma due to sarcoidosis. (B) Two months after steroid therapy, the granuloma and disc edema are resolving.

stage may present with peripheral anterior synechiae and secondary intraocular pressure elevation

Posterior segment involvement (14% to 20% of patients with ocular sarcoid): vitreous snowballs; granulomas of the retina, choroid, and optic nerve (Figures 4-11A and 4-11B); perivenous sheathing occurring as a linear or segmental periphlebitis; irregular nodular granulomas along venules "candle-wax drippings" (Figure 4-12); retinal vascular occlusion may occur and lead to neovascularization and vitreous hemorrhage; cystoid macular edema is common

Testing

- Chest CT or x-ray: very sensitive in detecting intrathoracic changes common in sarcoidosis
- Labs: ACE and lysozyme testing are of low value
- Gold standard is biopsy of affected tissue with histopathological confirmation of non-caseating granuloma formation
- Due to heterogenous presentation, a broad infectious and inflammatory workup should be performed to rule out other conditions that sarcoidosis may mimic.

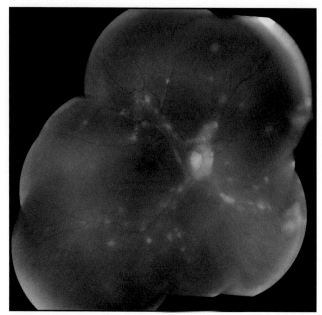

Figure 4-12. Ocular sarcoidosis. Color fundus photo with perivenous sheathing and irregular nodular granulomas ("candle-wax drippings"). (Reprinted with permission from Christopher Brady, MD.)

Differential Diagnosis

Infectious—syphilis, tuberculosis, Lyme disease; inflammatory—HLA-B27 associated uveitis, systemic lupus erythematosus, sympathetic ophthalmia (SO), Vogt-Koyanagi-Harada disease, Behçet's disease, polyarteritis nodosa, granulomatosis with polyangiitis (formerly Wegener's granulomatosis)

Management

- Corticosteroids are mainstay of treatment (topical, periocular, intravitreal and systemic)

- Systemic immunomodulating agents can be helpful including methotrexate, azathioprine, mycophenolate mofetil, cyclosporine, or TNF-α inhibitors

Behçet's Disease

Paul S. Baker, MD

- Systemic vasculitis with classic triad of oral ulcers (most common, 98%), genital ulcers, and uveitis. Most common in young adults 25 to 35 years old.
- Ocular involvement is usually bilateral (80% to 90%) with a relapsing and remitting course.
- Greatest incidence in Middle and Far East, particularly Japan and Turkey. Rare in the United States (0.2% to 0.4% of uveitis cases).

Signs and Symptoms

Decreased vision, pain, red eye, photophobia

Exam Findings

- Anterior: uveitis ranges from non-granulomatous anterior uveitis (with or without hypopyon) to panuveitis; conjunctivitis, scleritis, keratitis have been reported
- Posterior: retinal vasculitis of arteries and veins (most common), perivascular sheathing with exudates, deep retinal exudation, retinal necrosis, venous engorgement, capillary non-perfusion, secondary neovascularization, retinal detachment, vitritis, optic disc edema (Figure 4-13)
- End-stage disease is a blind, painful eye with neovascular glaucoma
- Systemic features: oral ulcers, painful or painless genital ulcers, skin disease (erythema nodosum, superficial thrombophlebitis, pyoderma, eruptions resembling acne vulgaris),

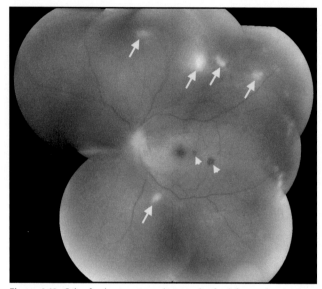

Figure 4-13. Color fundus montage photograph of a left eye showing hazy media due to vitritis, optic disc edema, perivascular sheathing, intraretinal hemorrhages (arrowheads), and scattered foci of retinitis (arrows).

arthritis (asymmetric, non-deforming, large joint polyarthritis), vascular disease (migratory superficial thrombophlebitis, thrombosis, arterial aneurysms)

- CNS disease due to vasculitis (eg, meningoencephalitis) carries greatest mortality; cranial nerve palsies can be observed

Testing

- Diagnosis is based on clinical criteria with no confirmatory lab testing.
- International study group: recurrent oral ulceration plus 2 of following: recurrent genital ulcers, uveitis, skin lesions, positive pathergy test

- HLA-B51 phenotype: present > 50% of Behçet's disease patients of Mediterranean and Japanese descent
- Pathergy skin reaction/Behcetine skin test (sterile pustule develops on skin at site of needle stick) is present in 40% of patients
- FA helps identify retinal vasculitis and non-perfusion
- MRI and CT scans with contrast may identify CNS lesions

Differential Diagnosis

Viral retinitis, HLA-B27 uveitis, syphilis, sarcoidosis, tuberculosis, systemic lupus erythematosus, polyarteritis nodosa, granulomatosis with polyangiitis

Management

Aggressive immunosuppression is critical. Systemic medication based on disease severity: pulse dose oral or IV corticosteroids have rapid anti-inflammatory effect. After initial disease control, immunosuppressive therapy for 12 to 18 months is usual before tapering. Steroid sparing agents are usually needed for long-term control: TNF inhibitors (infliximab and adalimumab), cytotoxic agents (chlorambucil, cyclophosphamide), anti-metabolites (azathioprine, mycophenolate mofetil), calcineurin inhibitors (cyclosporine, tacrolimus).

- Ocular: ocular steroids as needed to treat uveitis; laser photocoagulation and/or intravitreal anti-VEGF for neovascularization
- Anti-inflammatory treatment improves prognosis, but visual outcomes still very poor. In one series, legal blindness in > 50% of patients within 4 years.

Vogt-Koyanagi-Harada Disease

Sean T. Garrity, MD and
Andre J. Witkin, MD

- Multisystem inflammatory disorder targeting melanocytes, characterized by bilateral granulomatous panuveitis and serous retinal detachments (RD)
- More prevalent in darkly pigmented races

Signs and Symptoms

Prodromal phase (precedes ocular findings): headache, meningismus, tinnitus, dysacusis, flu-like symptoms, low-grade fever; acute uveitic phase: decreased vision, photophobia, pain, red eye, typically bilateral; convalescent phase: decreased vision; chronic recurrent phase: decreased vision, photophobia, pain, red eye

Exam Findings

- Anterior segment: anterior chamber cells and flare, granulomatous keratic precipitates, iris nodules, peripheral anterior or posterior synechiae, scleritis, hypotony or increased intraocular pressure
- Posterior segment: bilateral serous RD with choroidal thickening, vitreous cells and opacities, optic disc edema, mottling and atrophy of the RPE after resolution of RD (sunset glow fundus), retinal vasculitis, CNV, Dalen-Fuchs nodules (small, depigmented nodules beneath the retinal pigment epithelium)
- Systemic: vitiligo (blotchy loss of skin color), alopecia, poliosis (patch of white hair)

Testing

- FA:
  - Acute uveitic phase: multifocal areas of pinpoint hyper-fluorescence with late leakage, late staining of the disc, and pooling in areas of exudative detachment (Figure 4-14)
  - Convalescent phase: window defects due to RPE changes after resolution of subretinal fluid, staining in areas of fibrotic scarring
- ICGA: hypocyanescent dark dots, patchy delayed choroidal filling, hypercyanescent disc, stromal vessel hypercyanescence in early phase and indistinct borders of large stromal vessels in the intermediate phase
- OCT: subretinal fluid in areas of exudative detachment, thickened choroid during acute uveitic phase (Figure 4-15A)
- B-scan ultrasound: choroidal thickening with low to medium reflectivity, overlying retinal detachment, mild vitreous opacities, and posterior scleral thickening
- Lumbar puncture: cerebrospinal fluid analysis demonstrates pleocytosis in 84% of patients early in the disease course and typically resolves with treatment

Differential Diagnosis

SO, posterior scleritis, primary intraocular lymphoma, central serous chorioretinopathy, APMPPE, sarcoidosis uveitis, uveal effusion syndrome, tubercular syndrome, malignant hypertension, syphilitic uveitis

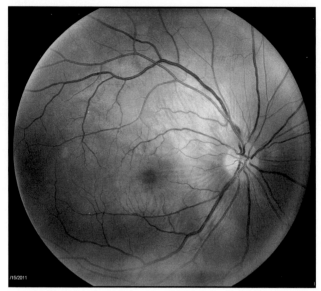

Figure 4-14. Acute uveitic phase: color fundus photo demonstrates subretinal, creamy-white lesions and areas of subretinal fluid.

Management

- Systemic corticosteroids—oral prednisone: 1.0 to 2.0 mg/kg once a day typically results in marked improvement in inflammation and resolution of exudative detachment within days
- Topical steroid and cycloplegic as adjuvant therapy. Immunomodulatory therapy—cyclosporine, azathioprine, methotrexate, cyclophosphamide, chlorambucil or mycophenolate mofetil are used if systemic steroids are inadequate in controlling the disease or patients develop intolerable side effects (Figures 4-15B and 4-15C).

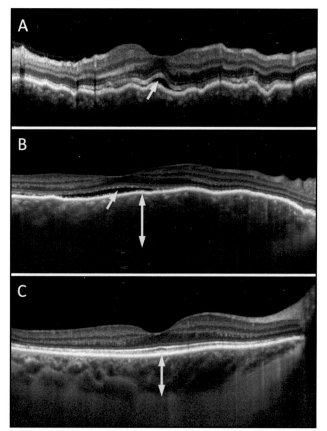

Figure 4-15. (A) OCT reveals pockets of subretinal fluid (arrow) in areas of exudative retinal detachment. (B) OCT after 2 weeks of systemic steroid therapy illustrates a shallow exudative retinal detachment (arrow) and thickened choroid (double arrow), which (C) resolved after 3 months of immunomodulatory therapy with mycophenolate mofetil.

Sympathetic Ophthalmia

Sean T. Garrity, MD and
Andre J. Witkin, MD

- Rare, bilateral, non-necrotizing granulomatous panuveitis that occurs after penetrating trauma or surgical insult to uvea of "exciting" eye. Pathogenesis of inflammation in fellow "sympathizing" eye is believed to result from ocular antigens in exciting eye being presented to systemic immune system.
- Usually asymmetric with more severe inflammation in exciting than sympathizing eye
- Onset can be acute or insidious, occurring months or years after injury, but most (90%) arise within a year of injury

Signs and Symptoms

Eye pain, photophobia, decreased vision, red eye, decreased accommodation (may be earliest symptom)

Exam Findings

Severe anterior chamber cells, large granulomatous keratic precipitates, Dalen-Fuchs nodules (small depigmented nodules beneath the retinal pigment epithelium; Figure 4-15), thickening of uveal tract (Figure 4-16). Additional findings may include peripheral anterior synechiae, iris neovascularization, occlusion and seclusion of pupil, cataract, exudative retinal detachment, and papillitis.

Testing

- FA:
  - Acute: multifocal areas of pinpoint hyperfluorescence with late leakage, late staining of the disc, and pooling in areas of exudative detachment

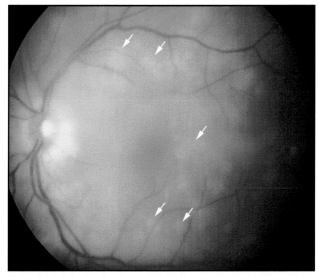

Figure 4-16. Color fundus photo of the left eye revealing moderate vitritis, multiple subretinal, creamy-white lesions (arrows), and peripapillary whitening.

- ◦ Chronic: window defects due to RPE changes, staining in areas of fibrotic scarring
- ICGA: choroidal inflammation during acute episodes, including hypocyanescent dark dots, patchy delayed choroidal filling, hypercyanescent disc, stromal vessel hypercyanescence in early phase and indistinct borders of large stromal vessels in intermediate phase
- OCT: subretinal fluid in areas of exudative detachment and thickened choroid during acute phase
- B-scan ultrasound: choroidal thickening with low to medium reflectivity, overlying retinal detachment, mild vitreous opacities, and posterior scleral thickening

Differential Diagnosis

Vogt-Koyanagi-Harada disease, sarcoidosis uveitis, tubercular syndrome, syphilitic uveitis, phacoanaphylactic endophthalmitis, posterior scleritis, primary intraocular lymphoma, central serous chorioretinopathy, APMPPE, uveal effusion syndrome, malignant hypertension

Management

- Preservative-free intravitreal Triesence (triamcinolone) has been approved by the Food and Drug Administration for SO
- Systemic steroids are useful to achieve rapid control, but if they are inadequate in controlling disease or intolerable side effects develop, steroid-sparing immunomodulatory therapy is required (eg, cyclosporine, azathioprine, methotrexate, cyclophosphamide, chlorambucil, and mycophenolate mofetil)
- Topical steroid and cycloplegic are adjuvant therapy
- Enucleation of a blind, traumatized, or disfigured eye within 14 days of trauma is recommended to prevent SO. However, once SO has developed the role for enucleation is unclear and remains controversial.

INTERMEDIATE UVEITIS (PARS PLANITIS)

Sundeep K. Kasi, MD

Typically affects children and young adults with bimodal peaks occurring between 5 to 15 years old and 25 to 35 years old. Testing to rule out associated autoimmune and infectious conditions is warranted for most patients; if workup is negative, a diagnosis of idiopathic pars planitis is typically made (70%).

Signs and Symptoms

Decreased vision, floaters; rarely associated with pain, photophobia, and redness

Exam Findings

Vitreous inflammatory cells (vitritis) and condensations of inflammation within vitreous (snowballs; Figure 4-17) or along vitreous base and pars plana (snowbanks), optic nerve edema, peripheral venous phlebitis, cystoid macular edema

Testing

- OCT: cystoid macular edema or retinal thickening
- FA: may demonstrate inflammation of macula, vessels, and optic nerve with petaloid macular edema and possible staining/leakage of vessel walls and optic nerve, peripheral non-perfusion
- Laboratory testing: CBC for evaluation of leukemia/lymphoma, erythrocyte sedimentation rate (ESR) and c-reactive protein (CRP) for evaluation of systemic inflammatory response, ACE and lysozyme for evaluation of sarcoidosis, RPR and FTA-ABS for evaluation of syphilis, QuantiFERON-TB Gold for evaluation of tuberculosis, and urinalysis (UA) for evaluation of tubulointerstitial nephritis and uveitis syndrome (TINU)
- Consider x-ray or CT of chest for evaluation of sarcoidosis and MRI of brain for evaluation in suspected cases of multiple sclerosis

Differential Diagnosis

Noninfectious causes: sarcoidosis (22%), multiple sclerosis, lymphoma, Blau syndrome, inflammatory bowel disease, TINU;

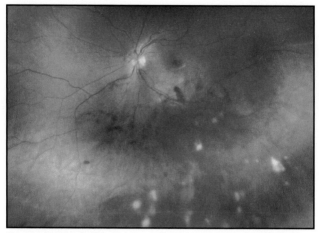

Figure 4-17. Wide-field fundus image demonstrating vitreous snowballs found in intermediate uveitis.

Infectious causes: tuberculosis, syphilis, Lyme disease, leprosy, toxocariasis, Whipple disease

Management

- Observation in mild cases with no symptoms and no macular edema
- Administration of corticosteroids initially: topical prednisolone or difluprednate, sub-Tenon's triamcinolone, intravitreal triamcinolone or Ozurdex (dexamethasone implant), oral prednisone
- Chronic and refractory inflammation: consider immunomodulatory therapies such as methotrexate, azathioprine, mycophenolate mofetil, tacrolimus, cyclosporine, infliximab, or adalimumab

- Laser for peripheral neovascularization due to inflammation (5% to 10%)
- Pars plana vitrectomy with or without laser to remove non-clearing vitreous debris or treat complications such as vitreous hemorrhage or retinal detachment (5%), or for diagnostic purposes

5

Retinal Degenerations and Dystrophies

RETINITIS PIGMENTOSA

Tomas S. Aleman, MD

- Molecularly heterogeneous group of inherited outer retinal degenerations that causes a bilateral, slowly progressive, pigmentary retinopathy
- Prevalence: Approximately 1:3500 and inherited in an autosomal recessive, dominant, or X-linked recessive pattern. Mitochondrial inheritance may exist in rare cases.
- Symptomatic onset typically in early adulthood although presentation can range from preschool years (early-onset retinal degenerations [EORDs]) to late adulthood (late-onset retinal degenerations [L-ORD])
- Syndromic retinitis pigmentosa (RP) distinguishes patients with confirmed or suspected systemic abnormalities (eg, sensorineural hearing loss, neurologic, and metabolic defects) from patients with only retinal disease [non-syndromic RP])

Hsu J, Chiang A, eds. *The Pocket Guide to Medical Retina* (pp 153-175).
© 2021 Taylor & Francis Group.

Signs and Symptoms

Nyctalopia, progressive visual field constriction, and eventually visual acuity loss; visual acuity is minimally impaired initially

Exam Findings

Initial grayish appearance of retinal pigment epithelium (RPE) with or without white spotted lesions; mid-peripheral, annular-like, pigmentary retinopathy later develops that expands both centripetally and centrifugally with age; waxy appearance to optic nerve and arteriolar attenuation with progression; vitreous cells may be present; end-stage disease characterized by diffuse pigmentary retinopathy with a depigmented or atrophic macula and total vision loss; posterior subcapsular cataracts in > 50%; cystoid macular edema (CME) may develop and epiretinal membranes are common (Figure 5-1A)

Testing

- Kinetic perimetry (Goldmann): mid-peripheral scotomas, generalized constriction with variable peripheral remnants of vision
- Color vision: preserved early on, tritan defects and multiple axis of confusion later in disease
- Short-wavelength fundus autofluorescence (AF) imaging: central islands of normal AF separated from peripheral regions of hypoautofluorescence by narrow hyperautofluorescence rings (Figure 5-1B)
- Optical coherence tomography (OCT): localized or diffuse photoreceptor outer segment loss and outer nuclear layer (ONL) thinning; total retinal thinning may be masked by a thickened inner retina due to remodeling (Figure 5-1C)
- Fluorescein angiography (FA): window defects from RPE loss; non-leaking CME; infrequently, choroidal neovascularization (CNV)

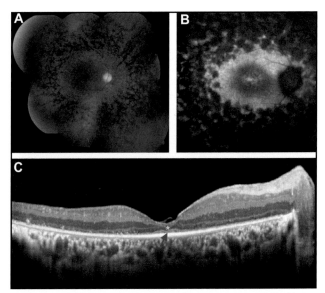

Figure 5-1. (A) Composite fundus picture of patient with typical RP showing bone spicule pigmentation in an annulus in the near mid-periphery. (B) Short-wavelength fundus AF shows signal limited to a central island with scalloped boundaries. (C) OCT cross-section through the fovea shows ONL thinning (*), loss of the outer retinal sublaminae (arrow), and overall retinal thinning.

- Electroretinography (ERG): abnormally reduced amplitudes with a rod > cone dysfunction

Differential Diagnosis

Cone dysfunctions and cone-rod dystrophies; congenital stationary night blindness, fundus albipunctatus, retinitis punctata albescens, severe Stargardt disease; choroidal dystrophies (choroideremia, gyrate atrophy, Bietti's crystalline dystrophy, central areolar and dystrophies, helicoidal); carrier state of inherited retinal degenerations (IRD; X-linked RP, choroideremia); hereditary vitreoretinopathies (familial exudative vitreoretinopathy,

Wagner and Stickler syndromes); autoimmune retinopathies; acute zonal occult outer retinopathy (AZOOR); post-infectious or post-inflammatory pigmentary retinopathies (pars planitis, birdshot chorioretinopathy, serpiginous retinopathy, multifocal placoid pigment epitheliopathy, sarcoidosis, rubella, syphilis, toxocara); vitamin A deficiency and abetalipoproteinemia; toxic retinopathies (thioridazine, chloroquine); neuro-ophthalmic diseases with inner retinal and visual field loss

Management

- Vitamin A palmitate: hyper-supplementation at 10,000 IU may slow progression; obtain clearance from primary care provider with monitoring for liver toxicity
- Docosahexaenoic acid (DHA): 400 mg by mouth 3 times a day
- Treatment of CME: topical and/or systemic carbonic anhydrase inhibitors (CAI) are first choice (eg, dorzolamide, brinzolamide); topical, periocular, or intravitreal steroids have a role if CAI and nonsteroidal anti-inflammatory drugs fail; anti-vascular endothelial growth factor (VEGF) injections may be used as a last resort
- Epiretinal electronic implants (Argus II [Second Sight]) approved by the Food and Drug Administration for end-stage disease with bare light perception or worse vision

CONE DYSTROPHIES

Tomas S. Aleman, MD

- Autosomal recessive and X-linked recessive patterns
- Stereotypical disease for this group of disorders is achromatopsia or total color blindness
- Incomplete forms: variable degree of residual cone function

  ◦ Blue cone monochromatism or rod monochromatism are X-linked subtype with preserved blue cone function
- Prevalence varies depending on molecular cause but is ~1:30,000 to 50,000

Signs and Symptoms

Typically present as infants or toddlers with nystagmus, photophobia and poor color discrimination and visual acuity; may also present later in life and into adulthood

Exam Findings

Fundus exam normal or blunted foveal reflex; may have small areas of depigmentation in and around foveal center; foveal atrophy occurs rarely (Figure 5-2A)

Testing

- Kinetic perimetry (Goldmann): fields mostly full or show mild generalized constriction
- Color vision: severely abnormal
- Full-field sensitivity testing (FST): normal rod-mediated sensitivities, severely abnormal cone vision
- Short-wavelength fundus AF imaging: preserved although may have central hypoautofluorescence in forms with more severe central disease (Figure 5-2B)
- OCT: foveal hypoplasia in some; foveal thinning with shortening and loss of the cone photoreceptor outer segment mainly at fovea (Figure 5-2C)
- ERG: normal rod function, cone ERGs are extremely reduced in amplitude to undetectable

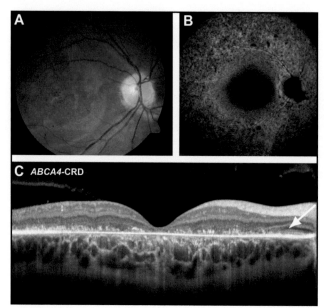

Figure 5-2. (A) Fundus photo of a patient with cone-rod dystrophy. (B) Near infrared AF demonstrating dense loss of RPE melanin centrally and diffuse loss into near mid-periphery. (C) Spectral domain-OCT vertical cross-section through the fovea shows severe ONL loss at the fovea with increased posterior backscattering and ONL preservation (arrow) in the peripapillary retina in this *ABCA4*-CRD patient.

Differential Diagnosis

Cone-rod dystrophies, Leber congenital amaurosis, neuronal ceroid lipofuscinoses, neuro-ophthalmic diseases with inner retinal and vision loss

Management

- Referral to comprehensive pediatric ophthalmologist for optimal correction of refractive errors, assessment of ocular alignment and amblyopia

- Referral to child development and educational specialists for early intervention and low vision rehabilitation
- Several promising gene therapy approaches are being tested (https://clinicaltrials.gov)

STARGARDT DISEASE

Tomas S. Aleman, MD

- Most frequent juvenile macular dystrophy with a prevalence of ~1:10,000 and onset typically in adolescence
- Typically autosomal recessive and associated with *ABCA4* gene mutations
- Onset and severity variable with milder forms showing adult onset and relative foveal preservation without atrophy termed *fundus flavimaculatus* (FFM)

Signs and Symptoms

Vision loss, impaired color vision

Exam Findings

Normal or blunted foveal reflex in early stages; variable central depigmentation and atrophy with a tapetal or beaten bronze sheen; pisciform whitish-yellow flecks distributed as an annulus around center and into mid-periphery which expand centripetally while most central lesions fade into central RPE atrophy (Figure 5-3A)

Testing

- Kinetic perimetry (Goldmann): fields are full peripherally with variable central scotomas depending on stage
- Static perimetry: central scotomas
- Color vision: normal in early disease, abnormal in later stages

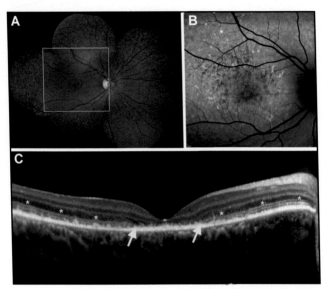

Figure 5-3. (A) Color fundus image of a patient with Stargardt disease showing characteristic yellow pisciform flecks. (B) Fundus AF showing areas of hypoautofluorescence in areas of RPE atrophy and hyperautofluorescence of flecks. (C) Spectral domain-OCT reveals loss of the ONL and ellipsoid zone (between arrows) in the fovea. The ONL (*) is intact outside the fovea.

- Short-wavelength fundus AF imaging: variable areas of hypoautofluorescence delineating areas of RPE atrophy (Figure 5-3B)
- OCT: foveal thinning early when fundus findings are minimal; overall retinal thinning with sharp transitions into normal appearing retina; distortion of photoreceptor-RPE interdigitation signal co-localizing with flecks (Figure 5-3C)
- FA: dark choroid typically with autosomal recessive Stargardt disease; flecks are hypofluorescent; window defects in areas of RPE atrophy
- ERG: normal rod and cone function, but in more advanced disease there may be reduction of both rod and cone

amplitudes; pattern of cone worse than rod dysfunction may be present in patients that are classified as cone-rod dystrophy

- Electrooculography (EOG): often abnormal

Differential Diagnosis

Cone-rod dystrophies, juvenile RP with macular involvement, syndromic RP, vitelliform macular dystrophies (atrophic stage), fundus albipunctatus, retinitis punctata albescens, neuronal ceroid lipofuscinoses, neuro-ophthalmic diseases with inner retinal and vision loss

Management

- Referral to comprehensive pediatric ophthalmologist for management of refractive errors, ocular alignment, and amblyopia
- Implantation of stem cell derived tissue is being studied as a treatment for patients with atrophic macular lesions

CONGENITAL STATIONARY NIGHT BLINDNESS

Tomas S. Aleman, MD

Large group of clinically and genetically heterogeneous, typically non-progressive retinal conditions with varying inheritance patterns (X-linked, autosomal recessive or autosomal dominant)

Signs and Symptoms

Nyctalopia and/or adaptation complaints; visual acuity usually preserved though some cases have reduced visual acuity; nystagmus, strabismus

Exam Findings

Normal fundus exam in most cases; flecks or white dots in retina can be seen in Oguchi disease and fundus albipunctatus

Testing

- Kinetic perimetry (Goldmann): fields are mostly full or minimally depressed
- OCT: foveal hypoplasia in some, inner retinal changes including nerve fiber layer loss and optic nerve atrophy reported in some specific genotypes
- Short-wavelength fundus AF imaging: preserved though there may be central hypoautofluorescence if more severe central disease is present
- ERG: reduced to undetectable rod responses and abnormal inner retinal response to maximal stimulation leading to a negative configuration ERG (Figure 5-4); abnormalities in outer retina may be present as well

Differential Diagnosis

Cone-rod dystrophies, Leber congenital amaurosis, X-linked retinoschisis, vitamin A deficiency, intraocular foreign body, ischemic retina, ocular albinism (OA), neuronal ceroid lipofuscinoses, neuro-ophthalmic diseases with inner retinal and vision loss

Management

- Referral to comprehensive pediatric ophthalmologist for optimal correction of refractive errors, assessment of ocular alignment and amblyopia
- Several promising gene therapy approaches are being tested (https://clinicaltrials.gov)

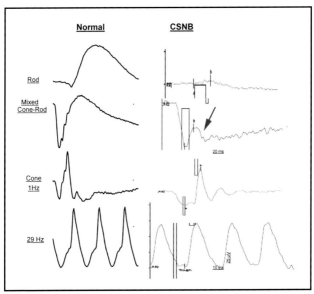

Figure 5-4. Standard electroretinogram in a patient with congenital stationary night blindness compared to a normal subject. Rod responses are reduced in amplitudes, combined rod-cone responses show a reduced b-wave (negative ERG; arrow), delayed cone ERGs.

VITELLIFORM MACULAR DYSTROPHY

Tomas S. Aleman, MD

- Hereditary retinal degeneration typically with a single (or sometimes multiple), oval, yellow subretinal macular deposit that can evolve into central chorioretinal atrophy
- Best disease: autosomal dominant vitelliform macular dystrophy (VMD) caused by mutations in *VMD2* that typically presents in adolescents or young adults

Signs and Symptoms

Visual acuity variably affected with good reading vision often into sixth decade

Exam Findings

Vitelliform lesions (typically macular but may be multifocal) of variable appearance that eventually evolve into atrophy (Figure 5-5A); macular lesions go through classic stages of vitelliform, pseudohypopyon, scrambled egg appearance to atrophy; secondary CNV

Testing

- Kinetic perimetry (Goldmann): fields are mostly full except in retina-wide presentations; central scotomas are expected
- Static perimetry: central scotomas
- Short-wavelength fundus AF imaging: central hyperautofluorescence (Figure 5-5B); central hypoautofluorescence in atrophic lesions
- OCT: elevated retina above a hyperreflective subretinal lesion with subretinal hyporeflective areas and variable degree of intraretinal hyporeflective spaces (Figure 5-5C); foveal atrophy in later stages; OCT angiography may show CNV
- FA: hyperfluorescence with passive leakage into lesions and some staining of the vitelliform lesions; window defects in atrophic lesions
- EOG: abnormal to undetectable in classic Best disease; normal EOG does not exclude disease (*VMD2*-associated disease)

Differential Diagnosis

Cone-rod dystrophies; adult-onset vitelliform dystrophy

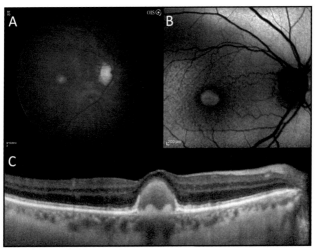

Figure 5-5. (A) Color fundus photo demonstrating a typical vitelliform lesion and surrounding small drusen. (B) Fundus AF shows central hyperautofluorescence. (C) OCT shows a subfoveal hyperreflective lesion elevating the retina. (Reprinted with permission from Jason Hsu, MD.)

Management

- Treatment of secondary CNV with intravitreal anti-VEGF therapy
- There is strong proof of concept for gene therapy as an option and clinical trials are in the planning stages.

PATTERN DYSTROPHIES

Tomas S. Aleman, MD

- Heterogeneous group of hereditary conditions characterized by bilateral, slowly progressive, mostly central, primarily RPE abnormalities

- Specific distributions of linear and/or dotted pigmentary changes have been used to sub-classify these conditions mainly as butterfly-shaped and reticular dystrophy; overlap with vitelliform, flecked and atrophic lesions

Signs and Symptoms

Metamorphopsia and/or blurred vision; visual acuity minimally impaired initially with slow progressive vision loss

Exam Findings

Central yellowish lesions with radial patterns or spotty yellow lesions (Figure 5-6A); grayish or darker appearance of RPE above lesions; flecks or drusen-like lesions surrounding main central lesion may form; pigment epithelial detachments and vitelliform lesions may be present; geography atrophy late in disease; CNV may develop

Testing

- Kinetic perimetry (Goldmann): usually normal peripheral extent; central and pericentral scotomas
- Color vision: preserved early on, multiple axis of confusion later
- Short-wavelength fundus AF imaging: linear hyperautofluorescence lesions surrounding central hyperautofluorescence image; hypoautofluorescence in areas of atrophy (Figure 5-6B)
- OCT: localized elevations of RPE band over a hyperreflective signal (Figure 5-6C); linear hyperreflective lesions tracking into ONL; local disruptions of photoreceptor outer segment signal; subretinal fluid in some cases; normal appearing retina interspaced between abnormal regions
- FA: window defects from RPE loss; infrequently, CNV
- ERG: normal or borderline reduced amplitudes
- EOG: normal or mildly reduced

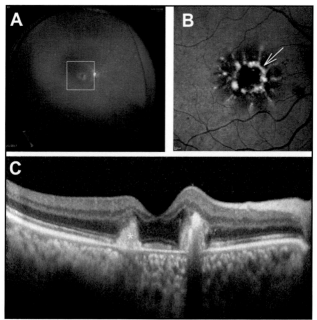

Figure 5-6. (A) Wide-angle fundus image of patient with pattern dystrophy. (B) Near infrared fundus AF in this patient showing ring with spoke pattern of hyperautofluorescence (arrow) that colocalizes with (C) elevations (*) of the RPE over a hyperreflective signal on spectral domain-OCT.

Differential Diagnosis

Stargardt disease, Best disease, cone-rod dystrophy, choroidal dystrophies (carrier states, central areolar dystrophies), carrier state of IRD (X-linked RP, choroideremia), medication induced (eg, deferoxamine)

Management

- Intravitreal anti-VEGF injections for CNV

- Discontinuation of offending drug should one be identified for secondary cases

CHOROIDEREMIA

Tomas S. Aleman, MD

- Molecularly homogeneous X-linked recessive inherited chorioretinal degeneration caused by mutations in REP1
- Prevalence is approximately 1:50,000 males
- Female carriers are usually asymptomatic but show various degree of localized pigmentary change often visible within central retina

Signs and Symptoms

Symptomatic onset typically in adolescence with nyctalopia followed by progressive visual field constriction; visual acuity usually declines by sixth decade

Exam Findings

Posterior subcapsular cataracts (>50%); vitreous syneresis; optic nerve pallor in late stages; bilateral, chorioretinal degeneration with white sclera visible through areas of scalloped chorioretinal atrophy or depigmented RPE with preservation of central island of retina by second to third decade of life (Figure 5-7A); dark patches representing remnants of RPE and retina in periphery by fourth decade; bone spicules less frequent and much less prominent than in RP; total chorioretinal atrophy late

Testing

- Kinetic perimetry (Goldmann): mid-peripheral scotomas, generalized constriction with variable peripheral remnants of vision

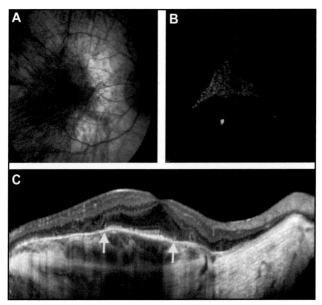

Figure 5-7. (A) Fundus photo showing visualization of the large choroidal vasculature and sclera through a depigmented RPE as well as a central island of relatively preserved RPE. (B) Short-wavelength fundus AF shows residual central island of fundus AF. (C) Horizontal spectral domain-OCT cross-section shows abrupt transition in thickness (outside of arrows) with ONL thinning, loss of the outer retinal sublaminae, and severe overall retinal thinning with increased posterior backscattering.

- Color vision: preserved early on, tritan defects and multiple axis of confusion later
- Short-wavelength fundus AF imaging: central islands of normal AF surrounded by peripheral regions of hypo AF (Figure 5-7B)
- OCT: localized or diffuse photoreceptor outer segment loss and ONL thinning early (Figure 5-7C); characteristic transitions between total retinal and choroidal thinning and normal appearing retina

- FA: window defects from RPE loss; CNV
- ERG: abnormally reduced amplitudes with rod > cone dysfunction, often becomes undetectable

Differential Diagnosis

RP or carrier state; choroidal dystrophies (gyrate atrophy → increased serum ornithine levels, end-stage Bietti's crystalline dystrophy, helicoidal); Sjögren reticular dystrophy, Leber congenital amaurosis, Kearns-Sayre syndrome, end-stage pattern dystrophy, end-stage Stargardt disease, retinal toxicity (thioridazine, pentosan polysulfate sodium)

Management

- Gene therapy currently in clinical trials with encouraging preliminary results
- Vitamin A palmitate 10,000 IU/day has been used but role not well-established
- Epiretinal electronic implant (Argus II [Second Sight]) for end-stage disease

OCULAR AND OCULOCUTANEOUS ALBINISM

Tomas S. Aleman, MD

- Non-progressive genetic disorders with reduced pigmentation of skin, hair and eye (oculocutaneous albinism [OCA]) or hypopigmentation of eye with minimal or no skin changes (OA)
- Autosomal recessive (OCA) and X-linked recessive (OA)
- Prevalence ~1:5000 to 17,000, depending on geographic region
- Variably impaired development of retina (foveal hypoplasia) and/or visual pathways (misrouting or greater crossing of temporal nerve fibers)

- Syndromic forms of OCA include Hermansky-Pudlak syndrome (hematologic and pulmonary disorders) and Chédiak-Higashi syndrome (immunologic abnormalities)

Signs and Symptoms

Visual acuity frequently abnormal to varying degrees

Exam Findings

Nystagmus, strabismus, iris transillumination often seen, visible choroidal vasculature through a depigmented fundus (Figure 5-8A), foveal hypoplasia

Testing

- Kinetic perimetry (Goldmann): may be difficult to perform due to photophobia but should be normal or show minimal peripheral depressions
- Color vision: usually normal or with nonspecific axis of confusion
- OCT: various degree of foveal hypoplasia (Figure 5-8B)
- ERG: normal
- Pattern visual evoked potential: demonstrates misrouting

Differential Diagnosis

Infantile nystagmus, achromatopsia and blue cone monochromatism, early-onset retinal dystrophies and Leber congenital amaurosis, neurologic causes of nystagmus in patients with fair complexion, albinoidism

Management

- Monitor ocular alignment early in life and offer proper rehabilitation and refraction

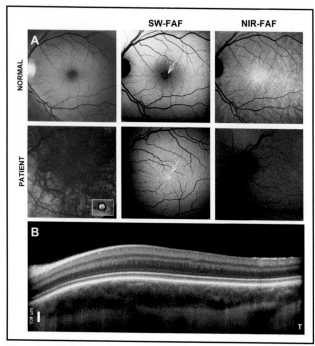

Figure 5-8. (A) Color fundus picture (inset is anterior segment picture), short wavelength and near infrared fundus AF in a patient with syndromic OCA (Hermansky-Pudlak syndrome associated with mutations in *HPS1*) compared to normal imaging. There is an expected brighter short-wavelength fundus AF signal near the foveola (arrows) compared to normal. There is hypoautofluorescent signal on near infrared fundus AF compared to normal. (B) Spectral domain-OCT horizontal section through position of anatomical fovea shows foveal hypoplasia with a flat foveal contour.

- Skin care is important as is protection from light with appropriate filters; early referral to a dermatologist is recommended
- Gene therapy is being considered experimentally

Autoimmune Retinopathies

Tomas S. Aleman, MD

- Inflammatory-mediated conditions characterized by acute (<3 months) or subacute (3 to 6 months) onset of progressive visual symptoms in association with serum anti-retinal antibodies (ARA) and a deceptively normal exam
- Paraneoplastic (pAIR) if preceding, during or following a diagnosis of a non-ocular cancer. Examples: cancer associated retinopathy (CAR) and melanoma associated retinopathy (MAR).
- Non-paraneoplastic (npAIR) if no association with cancer; overlaps with IRD

Signs and Symptoms

Photopsias, scotoma, dyschromatopsia, nyctalopia, photoaversion; visual acuity, visual fields, and color vision variably affected; may progress rapidly

Exam Findings

Normal fundus exam at presentation, CME has been described, absence of overt intraocular inflammation

Testing

- Kinetic perimetry (Goldmann): central or pericentral scotomas and variable overall depression of the fields

- Color vision: normal to abnormal (tritanopia, not definite axis)
- OCT: photoreceptor outer segment loss
- Short-wavelength fundus AF imaging: preserved but central, pericentral and peripapillary hypoautofluorescence lesions may be present
- ERG: reduced to undetectable rod responses and abnormal inner retinal responses to maximal stimulation leading to a negative configuration resembling congenital stationary night blindness in some cases (such as MAR; Figure 5-9); reduced rod- and cone-mediated ERGs that may progress to undetectable in forms of CAR
- Multifocal ERG: may show regional pericentral and/or central depressions
- Testing for presence of ARA

Differential Diagnosis

IRD, drug toxicity, ischemic retina

Management

- Comprehensive search for occult malignancies should occur promptly
- No randomized, placebo-controlled trials but following treatments have yielded variable results: steroids (local and systemic), conventional immunosuppression (eg, antimetabolites, T-cell inhibitors), biologics (eg, monoclonal antibodies), intravenous immunoglobulin (IVIg), plasmapheresis

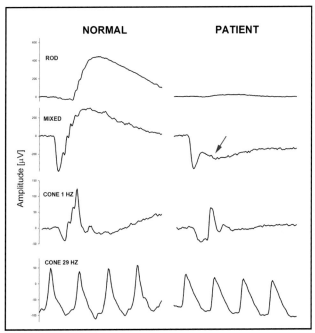

Figure 5-9. Standard electroretinogram in a patient with MAR compared to a normal subject. Rod responses are reduced in amplitudes, combined rod-cone responses show a reduced b-wave (negative ERG, arrow), and cone ERGs are delayed.

6

Pediatric Retinal Diseases

RETINOPATHY OF PREMATURITY

Turner D. Wibbelsman, BS and
James F. Vander, MD

- Leading cause of subsequent blindness and visual impairment in low birth weight and premature infants
- Associated with incomplete retinal vascular formation and secondary retinal neovascularization
- Systematic screening based on risk factors is critical
- Risk Factors: birth weight < 1500 g or gestational age < 30 weeks; birth weight 1500 to 2000 g or gestational age > 30 weeks with unstable clinical course

Exam Findings

Location (zone), extent (clock hours), stage, and plus disease status

Hsu J, Chiang A, eds. *The Pocket Guide to Medical Retina* (pp 177-198).
© 2021 Taylor & Francis Group.

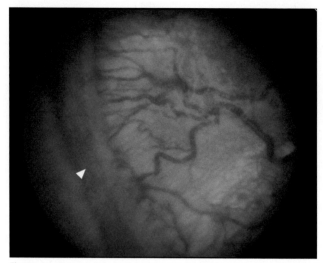

Figure 6-1. Stage 3 retinopathy of prematurity indicated by the extraretinal fibrovascular proliferation (arrowhead).

- Location: zone I—circle, radius of which extends from center of optic disc to twice the distance from center of optic disc to center of the macula; zone II—extends from edge of zone I to nasal ora serrata; zone III—residual crescent of retina anterior to zone II

- Stages: Stage 1—thin demarcation line separates vascular/avascular regions in peripheral retina; Stage 2—ridge with height and width separates vascular/avascular regions in peripheral retina; Stage 3—extraretinal fibrovascular proliferation or neovascularization from ridge into vitreous; Stage 4—(a) partial retinal detachment (RD), non-fovea involving and (b) partial RD, fovea involving; Stage 5—total RD (Figures 6-1 and 6-2)

- Pre-plus disease: more vascular engorgement and arterial tortuosity in posterior pole than normal

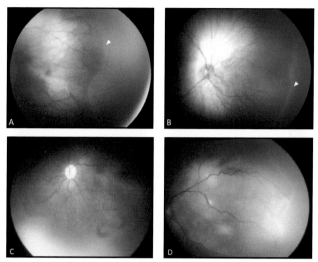

Figure 6-2. RetCam photographs of various retinopathy of prematurity disease stages. (A) Demarcation line (arrowhead) in Stage 1. (B) Ridge (arrowhead) in Stage 2 disease. (C) Zone I extraretinal fibrovascular proliferation in Stage 3. (D) Zone II extraretinal fibrovascular proliferation in Stage 3. (Reprinted with permission from Michael A. Klufas, MD.)

- Plus disease: 2 or more quadrants of vascular engorgement and arterial tortuosity in posterior pole (Figure 6-3)
- Involutional sequelae include tractional dragging, usually temporally, of major retinal vessels (Figure 6-4)

Testing

Telemedicine applications are currently being explored for large-scale screening efforts.

Differential Diagnosis

Family exudative vitreoretinopathy (FEVR), persistent fetal vasculature (PFV), RD, incontinentia pigmenti, Norrie

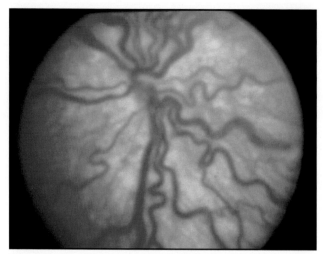

Figure 6-3. Plus disease in patient with retinopathy of prematurity. Arterial tortuosity and vascular engorgement are apparent.

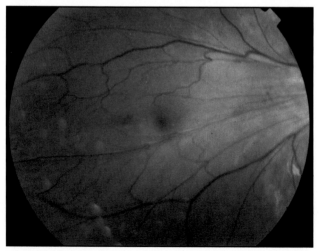

Figure 6-4. Dragged retinal vessels in patient with retinopathy of prematurity.

disease, shaken baby syndrome, X-linked retinoschisis, ocular toxocariasis, Coats disease, intermediate uveitis, endophthalmitis, retinoblastoma

Management

- Spontaneous regression in 85% of infants with Stage 1 retinopathy of prematurity (ROP)
- Confluent laser photocoagulation to avascular retina: indicated for zone I any stage with plus disease or Stage 3 without plus disease and zone II Stage 2 to 3 with plus disease
- Anti-vascular endothelial growth factor (VEGF) therapy: early evidence for benefit in zone I disease; long-term recurrence rate and systemic safety are yet to be determined
- Vitrectomy and/or scleral buckle: indicated for Stages 4 and 5 ROP; poor visual outcomes are common in these cases

FAMILIAL EXUDATIVE VITREORETINOPATHY

Samir Patel, MD and
Allen C. Ho, MD, FACS

- Rare, typically bilateral, inheritable disorder of retinal vascular development characterized by peripheral retinal nonperfusion and neovascularization
- Positive family history in 20% to 40% of cases with multiple modes of inheritance and variable expressivity: autosomal dominant (most common), autosomal recessive, X-linked recessive
- Nearly 50% of cases are linked to 4 causative genes (Norrie disease protein [NDP], Frizzled-4 [FZD4], low-density lipoprotein receptor-related protein 5 [LRP5], and tetraspanin-12 [TSPAN12]) that forms part of the Wnt signaling pathway

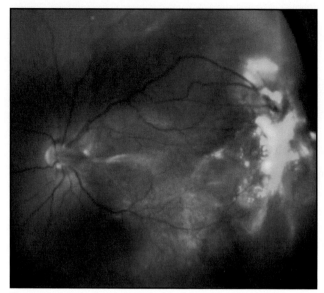

Figure 6-5. Color fundus photograph of the left eye showing temporal vascular dragging with subretinal exudation.

Signs and Symptoms

Most asymptomatic with mild disease, blurred vision, strabismus or leukocoria in children if severe

Exam Findings

Typically bilateral with asymmetric findings; peripheral retinal changes including retinal ischemia, neovascularization, macular dragging, subretinal exudation, vitreoretinal traction, and tractional and/or exudative RD (Figure 6-5)

- Proposed classification: Stage 1—avascular retinal periphery (a) without exudate (b) with exudate; Stage 2—retinal neovascularization (a) without exudate (b) with exudate; Stage 3—extramacular RD (a) without exudate (b)

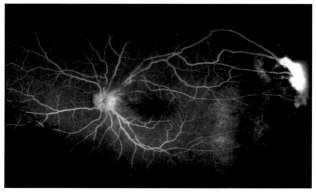

Figure 6-6. Ultra wide-field fluorescein angiogram of the left eye showing peripheral non-perfusion temporally with areas of hyperfluorescence and leakage corresponding to retinal neovascularization.

with exudate; Stage 4—macular involving RD, subtotal (a) without exudate (b) with exudate; Stage 5—total RD

Testing

- Wide-field fluorescein angiography (FA) of the patient and family members (Figure 6-6)
- Genetic testing for FEVR-related genes

Differential Diagnosis

ROP, incontinentia pigmenti, Eales disease, Coats disease, PFV, Norrie disease

Management

- Stage 1: typically requires no treatment but regular follow-up
- Stage 2: laser photocoagulation to all peripheral avascular areas
- Stages 3 to 5: vitrectomy with or without scleral buckling

○ Anti-VEGF therapy may be helpful prior to surgery, but should not be used as monotherapy

- FEVR is a lifelong disease that can progress and requires long-term follow-up.

COATS DISEASE

Douglas R. Matsunaga, MD and
Carl H. Park, MD

- Idiopathic, non-hereditary exudative retinopathy
- Unilateral, typically young males (median age of 5 years old) > females (20% to 30%)

Signs and Symptoms

Decreased vision, strabismus, leukocoria

Exam Findings

Retinal telangiectasia (typically peripheral) with associated lipid exudation (Figure 6-7), cystoid macular edema, epiretinal membrane, exudative RD, secondary neovascular glaucoma in end-stage disease with severe exudative detachment, less common: macrocyst, neovascularization

Testing

- FA: hyperfluorescent telangiectasia, hypofluorescent blockage by exudates, capillary non-perfusion, pooling in subretinal space (Figure 6-8)
- B-scan ultrasound: exudative RD with scattered hyperechogenicity due to high lipid content within subretinal fluid
- Fine needle aspiration biopsy: in ambiguous cases concerning for retinoblastoma; this will show lipid-laden macrophages and cholesterol crystals

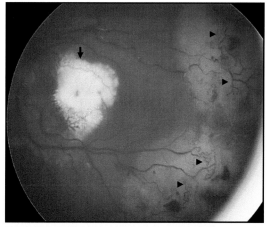

Figure 6-7. Fundus photograph demonstrating dense macular exudate (arrow), and extensive telangiectasia temporally (arrowheads). (Reprinted with permission from Carol L. Shields, MD.)

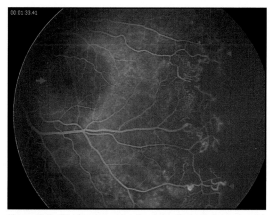

Figure 6-8. FA showing extensive telangiectasia (arrowheads), leakage and non-perfusion temporally (*), and macular hypofluorescent blockage (arrow) corresponding to dense exudate. (Reprinted with permission from Carol L. Shields, MD.)

Differential Diagnosis

Retinoblastoma, ROP, familial exudative vitreoretinopathy, retinal vasoproliferative tumor

Management

- Stable telangiectasia with no or minimal exudation (Stage 1): observation
- Telangiectasia with exudation (Stage 2): laser or cryotherapy
- RD (Stage 3): Pars plana vitrectomy (PPV) with laser photo-coagulation or cryotherapy. External drainage of subretinal fluid is an alternative to PPV.
- Total detachment and secondary glaucoma (Stage 4) with blind painful eye: consider evisceration/enucleation
- End-stage disease with phthisis bulbi (Stage 5) and non-painful blind eye: observation

CHORIORETINAL COLOBOMA

Phoebe L. Mellen, MD and
Ferhina S. Ali, MD, MPH

- Sporadic failure of embryonic fissure to close in the fifth week of development in utero
- May involve iris, lens, nerve, retina and retinal pigment epithelium (RPE)
- Usually inferonasal (typical coloboma), but can occur elsewhere

Signs and Symptoms

Poor vision if foveal involvement; scotoma if non-central involvement

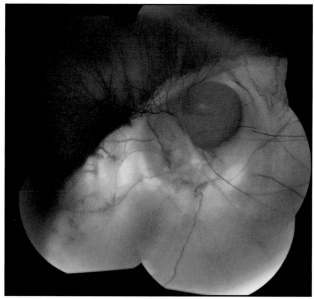

Figure 6-9. Fundus photograph of a large chorioretinal coloboma involving the optic nerve and extensive involvement of the posterior pole.

Exam Findings

Chorioretinal coloboma with whitening from lack of glial tissue and loss of RPE (Figure 6-9); pigmented demarcation line between absent and normal RPE; may be associated with RD or choroidal neovascularization (CNV); sectoral defect in upper eyelid (most common); flattening of lens equator, keyhole pupil from defects in iris tissue

Testing

Optical coherence tomography (OCT): atrophic retina, absent RPE, and choroid

Differential Diagnosis

Trauma, chorioretinal scar, staphyloma, morning glory disc, optic nerve pit, North Carolina macular dystrophy

Management

- Treat amblyopia and refractive errors
- Intravitreal anti-VEGF injections for CNV
- Vitrectomy for RD (chorioretinal coloboma increases the risk for RD)

Persistent Fetal Vasculature

Matthew Trese, DO, MA and
Cagri G. Besirli, MD, PhD

- Rare congenital disorder where tunica vasculosa lentis and/or hyaloid system do not regress
- Typically found in full-term healthy infants and is most commonly (~90%) unilateral

Categorization

- Anterior PFV: vascular stalk attached to posterior lens surface leading to cataract
- Posterior PFV: vascular stalk attached to optic nerve but not to posterior lens, may cause tractional RD (Figure 6-10A)
- Combined PFV: includes features of both anterior and posterior PFV, with one of these subtypes demonstrating predominance

Signs and Symptoms

Vision loss, leukocoria

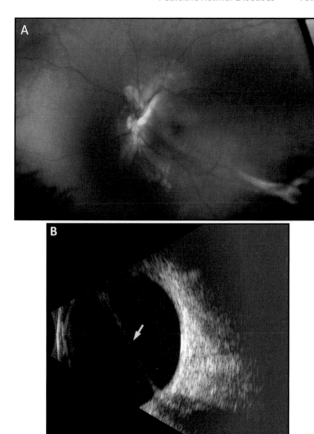

Figure 6-10. (A) Fundus photograph demonstrates posterior predominant PFV syndrome. (B) The stalk (arrow) is easily visualized using ultrasonography.

Exam Findings

Cataract, strabismus, elongated ciliary processes and a stalk on posterior surface of lens that may or may not extend to optic nerve; unilateral microphthalmia is common

Testing

- B-scan ultrasound or magnetic resonance imaging: visualize stalk if view of retina obscured by lens opacity (Figure 6-10B)
- Visual evoked potential (VEP): if signal present, may support more aggressive treatment in cases with traction RD
- FA and OCT: evaluate extent of retinal dysplasia, which may limit visual potential

Differential Diagnosis

Retinoblastoma, congenital cataract, ROP, Coats disease, ocular toxocariasis, Norrie disease, FEVR, incontinentia pigmenti

Management

- Surgical intervention often provides patients with best possible visual outcomes
  - If cataract is significant, lens should be removed and stalk transected to eliminate tractional forces on retina
  - In absence of significant cataract, a lens-sparing vitrectomy may be performed to divide posterior stalk

X-LINKED RETINOSCHISIS

Turner D. Wibbelsman, BS and
Michael A. Klufas, MD

- Hereditary disorder affecting mostly males bilaterally with prevalence of ~1:5000 to 25,000 males
- Linked to *RS1* gene on X chromosome (Xp22.1-p22.3) that encodes retinoschisin

Signs and Symptoms

Decreased vision (often detected at school age); less common: squint/nystagmus in early infancy, hyperopia more common than myopia

Exam Findings

Stellate macula (foveal retinoschisis with splitting at level of nerve fiber layer [NFL]) in young patients (Figure 6-11A); blunted foveal reflex, mild RPE abnormalities in older patients; peripheral retinoschisis in ~50% of patients, more common inferiorly; perivascular sheathing, microvascular abnormality, neovascularization; vitreous hemorrhage from rupture of unsupported retinal vessels; tractional or exudative RD; breaks may lead to rhegmatogenous RD (Figure 6-11B); elevated bullous retinoschisis with hemorrhage in schisis cavity

Testing

- OCT: area of retinoschisis extends through macula and up to vascular arcades; cystoid changes from retinal NFL to inner nuclear layer; thinning of NFL (Figure 6-11C)
- FA: no leakage in macula; RPE alterations in older males
- Electroretinography (ERG): selective loss of b-wave with normal a-wave, suggesting Müller cell dysfunction
- Genetic testing of patient and family as well as clinical examination of family members

Differential Diagnosis

Enhanced S-cone syndrome (Goldmann-Favre syndrome), ROP, familial exudative vitreoretinopathy, retinitis pigmentosa, Norrie disease, Stargardt disease, refractive/strabismic amblyopia

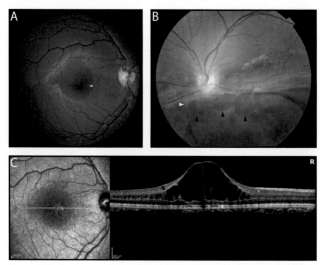

Figure 6-11. (A) Fundus photograph of stellate macula in patient with X-linked retinoschisis. Note the "spoke-wheel" pattern (arrowhead) of schisis in the fovea. (B) Fundus photograph with X-linked retinoschisis exhibiting retinal breaks (black arrows) and an unsupported vessel (white arrow) traversing the area of schisis. (C) Spectral domain OCT of foveoschisis prominently involving the NFL and inner retina.

Management

- Topical carbonic anhydrase inhibitors may improve retinal anatomy and visual function in some patients.
- Surgery: vitrectomy for persistent vitreous hemorrhage; vitrectomy and/or scleral buckle for RD (tractional or rhegmatogenous)

Early-Onset Severe Retinal Dystrophy and Leber Congenital Amaurosis

Tomas S. Aleman, MD

- Leber congenital amaurosis (LCA): heterogeneous group of inherited retinal degenerations that causes severe vision loss before 1 year of age
- Early-onset severe retinal dystrophy (EOSRD), early-onset retinal degeneration (EORD), severe early–childhood-onset retinal dystrophy (SECORD), childhood onset severe retinal dystrophy and juvenile retinitis pigmentosa, are used to classify conditions that overlap with LCA but present later in childhood
- Syndromic forms: Bardet-Biedl (obesity, polydactyly, cognitive impairment, genitourinary and renal abnormalities), Joubert (brain abnormalities, hypotonia, developmental delays), Meckel (renal cysts, central nervous system anomalies, hepatic abnormalities, and polydactyly), Senior-Løken (nephronophthisis), Conorenal (cone-shaped digital epiphyses and cerebellar hypoplasia)
- Autosomal recessive inheritance in vast majority of the cases with prevalence of ~2 to 3 per 100,000

Signs and Symptoms

Visual inattention, abnormal eye movements, difficulties ambulating, photophobia, nyctalopia, persistent staring at bright lights, eye poking (Franceschetti's oculo-digital sign)

Exam Findings

- Anterior segment: sluggish pupillary reactions in LCA; keratoconus may be associated (*CRB1-* and *AIPL1*-EOSRD); congenital cataracts; posterior subcapsular cataracts later

- Posterior segment: early on, fundus exam normal or limited to grayish appearance of RPE with or without white spotted lesions; later, pigmentary retinopathy develops with waxy appearance to optic nerve, arteriolar attenuation and retina-wide pigmentary changes (Figures 6-12A and 6-12B)

Testing

- Kinetic perimetry (Goldmann): fields undetectable in most LCA patients, severe generalized constriction with variable peripheral remnants of vision
- Color vision: undetectable to severely abnormal
- Pupillometry: insensitive pupil responses, participation of non-classical photoreceptors
- Full-field sensitivity testing (FST): sensitivity loss often in excess of 30 dB
- OCT: Localized or diffuse photoreceptor outer segment loss and outer nuclear layer thinning, which may be masked by a thickened inner retina due to remodeling. In some forms OCT may appear normal despite severe vision loss (*GUCY2D*-EOSRD; Figures 6-12C and 6-12D).
- Short-wavelength fundus autofluorescence (AF): Central islands of normal AF surrounded by peripheral regions of hypoautofluorescence. There may be central hypoauto-fluorescence in forms with predominant central disease or reduced to undetectable (*RPE65*-LCA).
- ERG: extremely reduced or undetectable amplitudes

Differential Diagnosis

Achromatopsia, cone-rod dystrophies, neuronal ceroid lipo-fuscinoses, peroxisomal biogenesis disorders (Zellweger syndrome, neonatal adrenoleukodystrophy, Infantile Refsum disease); hereditary vitreoretinopathies (familial exudative vitreo-retinopathy, Wagner and Stickler syndromes); neuro-ophthalmic

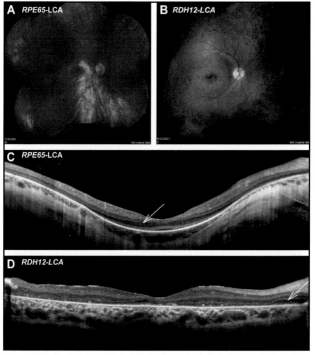

Figure 6-12. Composite fundus pictures of 2 patients representing 2 sides of the spectrum of LCA. (A) Relative central preservation (*RPE65*-LCA) vs (B) LCA with predominantly central disease (*RDH12*-LCA). (C) Spectral domain-OCT shows outer nuclear layer preservation (arrow) in the foveal/parafoveal region in *RPE65*-LCA. (D) In contrast, better preserved outer nuclear layer is observed in more eccentric peripapillary retina (arrow) in *RDH12*-LCA outer nuclear layer.

diseases with inner retinal and vision loss, abetalipoproteinemia, retinitis pigmentosa

Management

- Gene therapy approved by the Food and Drug Administration for subretinal delivery in *RPE65*-LCA (Luxturna [voretigene neparvovec-rzyl]) dramatically improves rod- and cone-mediated visual fields

- Several other promising gene therapy approaches are being tested

INCONTINENTIA PIGMENTI

Raymond Ko, MD, FRCSC, BSc and
Michael Dollin, MD, FRCSC

- Rare, X-linked dominant phakomatosis, also known as Bloch-Sulzberger syndrome
- Mutation in *IKBKG* gene detected in 80%
- Almost all affected are females with mother-daughter transmission in familial cases; lethal in hemizygous males

Signs and Symptoms

Vision loss may be severe, strabismus

Exam Findings

- Ocular (35%)—proliferative retinal vasculopathy: typically unilateral or markedly asymmetric; characterized by zones of peripheral avascularity, arterio-venous connections, neovascularization, and retinal hemorrhages (Figure 6-13); rapid progression may lead to tractional or exudative RD and retrolental membranes; cataract, foveal hypoplasia, optic hypoplasia or atrophy, nystagmus
- Dermatologic (100%)—progressive skin lesions: normal appearance at birth; erythematous bullae on arms and legs evolving to hyperpigmented macules appearing whorled or like "splashed-paint" weeks to months in infancy; patchy hypopigmentation with cutaneous atrophy in adults
- Dental (70%): missing and malformed teeth

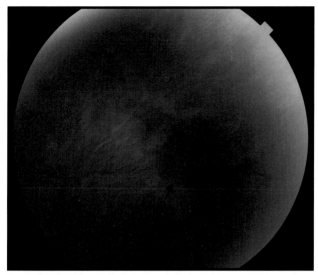

Figure 6-13. Peripheral retinal neovascularization with preretinal hemorrhage (arrow) in a patient with incontinentia pigmenti.

- Neurologic (30%): seizures and cognitive impairment most common

Testing

- FA: enlarged foveal avascular zone, peripheral hyperfluorescence with leakage from neovascularization, adjacent to hypofluorescent, avascular retina (Figure 6-14)
- OCT: inner retinal thinning and irregular outer plexiform layer
- OCT angiography: decreased vascular density, abnormal vascular loops, and flow loss in vascular plexuses

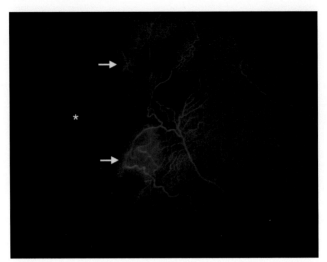

Figure 6-14. Fluorescein angiogram demonstrating avascular retina (*), and retinal vessel anastomoses and neovascularization (arrows) at the border between perfused and non-perfused retina.

Differential Diagnosis

ROP, familial exudative vitreoretinopathy, Norrie disease, Eales disease, sickle cell retinopathy

Management

- Laser photocoagulation or cryotherapy of avascular retina
- PPV with or without scleral buckle if RD
- Potential role for intravitreal anti-VEGF injections being investigated

7

Trauma-Related Retinopathies

Commotio Retinae

Musa Abdelaziz, MD and
Eric D. Weichel, MD

Self-limited opacification of retina secondary to direct blunt ocular trauma

Signs and Symptoms

Decreased vision, pain after recent trauma

Exam Findings

Retinal whitening in macula (Berlin's edema) and/or peripherally (Figure 7-1A); retinal, preretinal, and/or subretinal hemorrhages

Hsu J, Chiang A, eds. *The Pocket Guide to Medical Retina* (pp 199-218).
© 2021 Taylor & Francis Group.

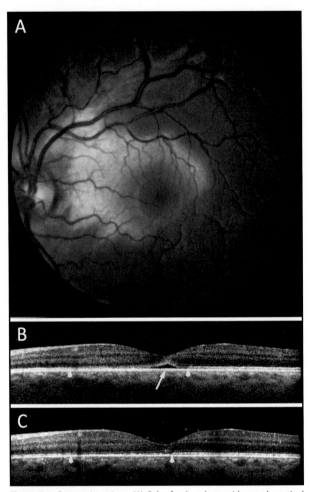

Figure 7-1. Commotio retinae. (A) Color fundus photo with macular retinal whitening consisted with Berlin's edema. (B) OCT of acute commotio showing abnormality of the ellipsoid zone (between arrowheads) and subretinal fluid (arrow). (C) One week later, OCT showed resolution of the subretinal fluid but attenuation of the ellipsoid zone (between arrowheads). (Reprinted with permission from William E. Benson, MD.)

Testing

Optical coherence tomography (OCT): early post-trauma hyperreflectivity of photoreceptor layers (ellipsoid zone), followed by thinning of photoreceptor layer (Figures 7-1B and 7-1C)

Differential Diagnosis

Choroidal rupture, chorioretinitis sclopetaria, traumatic retinal hole, Purtscher retinopathy

Management

No treatment is indicated or available, other than observation.

CHOROIDAL RUPTURE

Kevin Broderick, MD and
Eric D. Weichel, MD

Typically due to blunt trauma causing tears of choroid, retinal pigment epithelium (RPE), and Bruch's membrane

Signs and Symptoms

Decreased vision, metamorphopsia; asymptomatic if lesion is not involving central macula

Exam Findings

Yellow or white curvilinear subretinal streak(s) typically oriented in concentric pattern with disc margin often associated with subretinal hemorrhage, which may initially mask underlying rupture; hyperpigmentation at margins with chronicity; new hemorrhage or subretinal fluid if choroidal neovascularization (CNV) develops (Figure 7-2A)

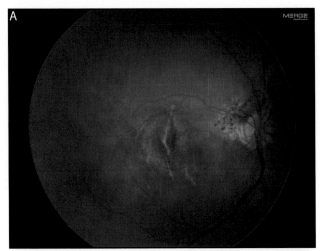

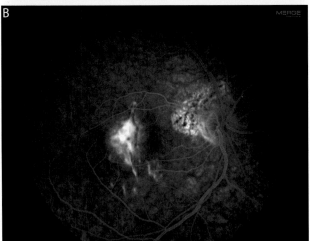

Figure 7-2. (A) Color fundus photograph showing choroidal rupture within the macula of a 16-year-old male who suffered blunt trauma to the right eye 1 month prior. (B) FA revealing late leakage adjacent to the choroidal rupture consistent with active CNV.

Testing

- OCT: discontinuity of Bruch's membrane, subretinal hyper-reflective material when subretinal hemorrhage present, subretinal fluid if CNV
- Fluorescein angiography (FA): may show leakage in acute setting from ruptured choroidal vasculature into retina; healed ruptures show early hypofluorescence within rupture and late hyperfluorescenct staining; if CNV, well-defined early hyperfluorescence with late leakage (Figure 7-2B)
- Fundus autofluorescence: hypoautofluorescence within rupture, hyperautofluorescence of rim around rupture, blocked autofluorescence when hemorrhage present

Differential Diagnosis

Angioid streaks, lacquer cracks

Management

- Isolated choroidal rupture(s): observation with regular monitoring and Amsler grid testing for detection of CNV
- CNV: intravitreal anti-vascular endothelial growth factor (VEGF) therapy is first-line treatment; laser photocoagulation if extrafoveal; photodynamic therapy

CHORIORETINITIS SCLOPETARIA

Turner D. Wibbelsman, BS and
Michael A. Klufas, MD

Results from high-velocity projectile (eg, pellet, BB, bullet) passing adjacent to globe near or in orbit without globe penetration causing concussive ("shock wave") forces

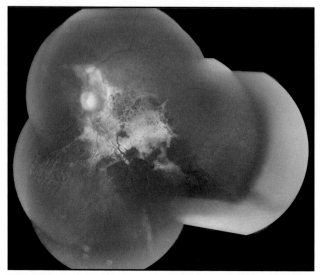

Figure 7-3. Retinal whitening and pigmented fibroproliferative tissues along with subretinal hemorrhage inferotemporally observed in eye with chorioretinitis sclopetaria.

Signs and Symptoms

Varying visual acuity depending on injury location and severity

Exam Findings

Full-thickness retinal and choroidal rupture, choroidal and retinal hemorrhages (sub-, intra- and preretinal), vitreous hemorrhage, healed rupture sites leave white, partially-pigmented fibroproliferative tissue (Figure 7-3)

Testing

- B-scan ultrasound: assess globe integrity for possible rupture
- Computed tomography (CT) scan: assist in locating projectile, identifying additional orbital injuries; thin (1 mm) cuts to rule out occult globe penetration/intraocular foreign body (IOFB)
- OCT: full-thickness rupture may appear hyperreflective

Differential Diagnosis

Ruptured globe, choroidal rupture, IOFB

Management

- Observation initially: fibroglial scarring can fuse retinal and choroidal tissue, decreasing chances of retinal detachment (RD)
- Consider topical steroids and/or topical cycloplegic for pain control/ciliary body spasm
- Vitrectomy if persistent vitreous hemorrhage or RD

AVULSION OF THE VITREOUS BASE

Ehsan Rahimy, MD

- Pathognomonic of previous ocular trauma
- Anteroposterior compression of globe during blunt ocular trauma leads to equatorial expansion which may avulse vitreous base from retina and pars plana
- More common in superonasal and inferotemporal quadrants

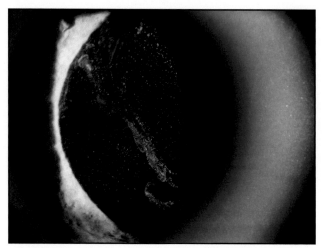

Figure 7-4. Curvilinear vitreous condensation characteristic of avulsed vitreous base with pigmented debris visible on slit lamp exam. (Reprinted with permission from William E. Benson, MD.)

Signs and Symptoms

Blurry vision, floaters, photopsias, progressive peripheral visual field defect if associated with a RD

Exam Findings

Curvilinear "bucket handle" vitreous condensation hanging over peripheral retina (Figure 7-4); if extensive, may be visible in anterior vitreous on slit lamp examination; potentially associated findings: iritis, angle recession, traumatic cataract, vitreous hemorrhage, anterior vitreous pigment, posterior vitreous detachment, commotio retinae, intraretinal hemorrhages, retinal breaks, retinal dialysis, RD

Differential Diagnosis

Retinal dialysis, peripheral RD

Management

Thorough peripheral exam with scleral depression along with close follow-up given high-risk of RD

PHOTIC INJURY

M. Ali Khan, MD

- Prolonged exposure to intense light source leads to release of reactive oxygen species
- Common causes: solar retinopathy, Welder's maculopathy, surgical illumination (operating microscope and/or endoilluminators), accidental hand-held laser injury
- Risk factors: young age, use of photosensitizing or illicit drugs, impaired mental status (prolonged sun gazing), clear intraocular lens

Signs and Symptoms

Decreased vision, central scotoma, erythropsia (reddish hue to vision)

Exam Findings

Focal, yellow-white foveal lesion which may fade with time (Figure 7-5); larger areas of retinal whitening or yellowing may be present with more widespread exposure; concurrent photo-keratitis; secondary findings: CNV, subretinal hemorrhage (Figure 7-6A), subhyaloid hemorrhage, macular hole, and epiretinal membrane may develop post injury

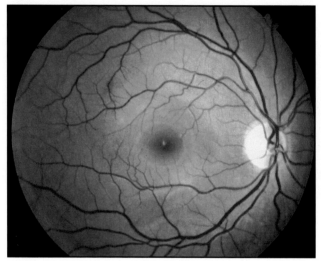

Figure 7-5. Fundus photo of solar retinopathy showing a focal yellowish foveal lesion.

Testing

- FA: may initially appear normal, but speckled areas of hyper- and hypofluorescence may be present in areas of RPE atrophy (Figure 7-6B)
- OCT: well-defined, outer retinal disruption of the photoreceptor layer/ellipsoid zone; hyperreflective vertical bands and hyporeflective cavities in the outer retina (Figure 7-6C)
- Autofluorescence: central hypoautofluorescence with a rim of hyperautofluorescence due to focal or diffuse RPE atrophy and mottling

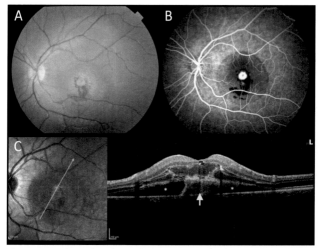

Figure 7-6. (A) Fundus photo of laser injury to fovea demonstrating hard exudates, subretinal fluid and subretinal hemorrhage. (B) FA shows central hyperfluorescence at the injury site with surrounding hypofluorescence from hemorrhage. (C) OCT confirms retinal thickening, disruption of the outer retinal layers, subfoveal hyperreflective material corresponding to exudation and hemorrhage (arrow), and surrounding hyporeflectivity from subretinal fluid (*).

Differential Diagnosis

Macular pseudohole, macular dystrophy, age-related macular degeneration, alkyl nitrate ("popper") related maculopathy, achromatopsia/rod monochromatism

Management

- Monitoring and treatment of any secondary CNV
- Risk mitigation: education, safety equipment, and regulatory standards

Valsalva Retinopathy

Hannah Levin, BS and
Jason Hsu, MD

- Unilateral or bilateral rupture of superficial retinal capillaries
- Secondary to an acute rise in intraocular venous pressure, due to increased intrathoracic pressure related to a strenuous physical act such as: aerobic exercise, lifting, sexual activity, constipation, surgical procedures, vomiting, coughing, pregnancy
- Risk factors include history of vascular disease and ocular venous occlusions

Signs and Symptoms

Sudden, painless loss of vision; central scotoma, may be asymptomatic

Exam Findings

Well-circumscribed or round preretinal hemorrhage(s) in macula beneath internal limiting membrane (ILM), but occasionally subhyaloid or intravitreous (Figures 7-7A and 7-7C)

Testing

- OCT: preretinal hyperreflectivity due to hemorrhage with overlying membrane (ILM and/or posterior hyaloid, fused or unfused; Figures 7-7B and 7-7D)
- B-scan ultrasound: evaluate for RD or tear if vitreous hemorrhage obscures view
- FA: rule out other causes of retinal hemorrhage

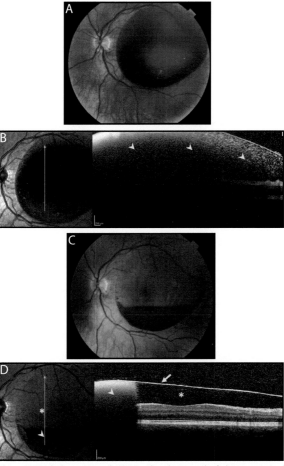

Figure 7-7. Valsalva retinopathy. (A) Fundus photograph of a large preretinal macular hemorrhage 2 weeks post-Valsalva stress. (B) Corresponding OCT shows sub-hyaloid/sub-ILM hemorrhage (arrowheads) obscuring the underlying retina. (C) At 6 weeks, hemorrhage is resolving and has settled into boat shape. (D) Corresponding OCT shows the preretinal hemorrhage layering inferiorly (arrowheads), the sub-ILM space (*), and the separated posterior hyaloid/ILM (arrow).

Differential Diagnosis

Retinal arterial macroaneurysm, diabetic retinopathy, hypertensive retinopathy, venous occlusion, anemia, retinal tear, posterior vitreous detachment

Management

- Observation as most cases resolve spontaneously
- If hemorrhage is not clearing in a timely manner, consider vitrectomy with removal of ILM or Nd:YAG laser to create opening in ILM for hemorrhage to escape

SHAKEN BABY SYNDROME

Connie M. Wu, MD and
Michael A. Klufas, MD

- Abusive head trauma resulting from internal acceleration and deceleration forces often without blunt head impact
- Usually bilateral (< 20% asymmetric, 2% unilateral) and signs of external trauma are not necessarily present
- Usually occurs in children < 1 year old, not common > 3 years old

Signs and Symptoms

New onset seizures, irritability, appetite or behavioral change, mental status change, ecchymosis, lethargy, developmental delay

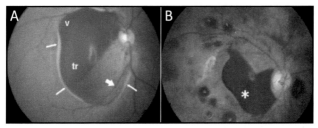

Figure 7-8. (A) Traumatic macular retinoschisis with retinal fold at edge of schisis (thin arrows), sub-ILM hemorrhage within the schisis cavity (tr) and vitreous hemorrhage (v). Note the vessel traveling up the schisis cavity and then down (thick arrow). (B) Numerous retinal hemorrhages throughout the posterior pole with preretinal/subhyaloid blood (*) but no evidence of retinal folds or retinoschisis. (Reprinted with permission from Alex V. Levin, MD, MHSc.)

Exam Findings

Retinal hemorrhages (all layers) in 85% (Figure 7-8), vitreous hemorrhage less common, hemorrhagic macular cysts in sub-ILM and/or macular schisis, associated fractures of ribs or long bones, subarachnoid and subdural intracranial hemorrhages

Testing

- B-scan ultrasound: useful when dense vitreous hemorrhage present
- OCT: detect retinoschisis and foveal disruption
- CT/magnetic resonance imaging of head and orbits to evaluate for intracranial hemorrhage, skeletal survey and/or bone scan
- Labs: complete blood count, prothrombin time/international normalized ratio, partial thromboplastin time; consider fibrinogen, D-dimer, clotting factor levels, von Willebrand factor

Differential Diagnosis

Birth trauma (especially with use of forceps delivery), blood dyscrasias (eg, leukemia), severe hypertension, ruptured intracranial aneurysm vs other hyperacute rise in intracranial pressure

Management

- Pediatric consultation to evaluate for child abuse and delayed neurological development
- Treat systemic findings (eg, fractures, brain trauma, associated complications)
- In rare cases of dense vitreous hemorrhage, consider vitrectomy if concern for amblyopia
- Prognosis largely depends on extent of any associated brain injury. Poor pupillary response, poor visual acuity, and retinal hemorrhages have been associated with high infant mortality.

TERSON'S SYNDROME

Jason Hsu, MD

- Intraocular hemorrhage, usually bilateral, related to spontaneous or trauma-induced intracranial hemorrhage
- Seen in ~20% with acute intracranial bleeding; only ~3-5% have significant vitreous hemorrhage
- Most common cause: subarachnoid hemorrhage from cerebral aneurysm

Signs and Symptoms

Blurred vision that varies depending on extent of intraocular hemorrhage

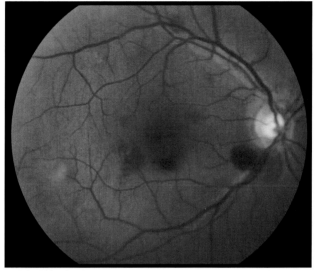

Figure 7-9. Color fundus photo demonstrating premacular hemorrhages characteristic of Terson's syndrome.

Exam Findings

Multiple, usually bilateral, retinal hemorrhages typically more superficial (eg, sub-ILM or subhyaloid; Figure 7-9); vitreous hemorrhage; late findings: epiretinal membrane, macular hole, perimacular retinal folds; rare findings: traction or rhegmatogenous RD

Testing

- B-scan ultrasonography: can be helpful to rule out RD if vitreous hemorrhage is present
- CT scan: evaluate for intracranial hemorrhage

Differential Diagnosis

Purtscher retinopathy, shaken baby syndrome, valsalva retinopathy, blood dyscrasia

Management

- Observation as hemorrhage may clear spontaneously
- Vitrectomy surgery: if non-clearing vitreous and/or preretinal hemorrhage, epiretinal membrane, or RD

PURTSCHER AND PURTSCHER-LIKE RETINOPATHY

Anthony Obeid, MD and
Carl D. Regillo, MD

- Categorized as either Purtscher retinopathy (when secondary to cranial or thoracic trauma) or Purtcher like-retinopathy (when associated with non-traumatic etiologies such as pancreatitis, pancreatic adenocarcinoma, renal failure, connective tissue disorders [systemic lupus erythematosus, scleroderma, dermatomyositis], embolism [fat, air, amniotic fluid], cryoglobulinemia, hemolytic urenic syndrome, thrombotic thrombocytopenic purpura, hemolysis/elevated liver enzymes/low platelets [HELLP] syndrome and pre-eclampsia)
- May result from precapillary arteriolar occlusion secondary to microembolization due to either fat embolization or complement activation with leukoaggregation
- Bilateral in ~60%

Signs and Symptoms

Vision loss (~54% of cases ≤20/200); central, paracentral, or arcuate scotomas; symptoms may be delayed by up to 24 to 48 hours

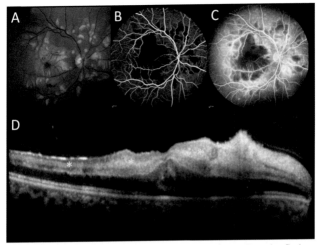

Figure 7-10. (A) Fundus photo with multiple cotton wool spots, Purtscher flecken, and a few retinal hemorrhages. (B) Mid-phase fluorescein angiogram showing blocked fluorescence corresponding to the retinal whitening. (C) Later-phase fluorescein angiogram showing staining of the retinal vessels and late leakage in areas of ischemia. (D) OCT demonstrating inner retinal hyperreflectivity (*) and macular edema.

Exam Findings

- Common findings: peripapillary or posterior pole cotton wool spots (~93%), retinal hemorrhages (~65%), and Purtscher flecken (polygonal whitening of inner retina that spares the areas immediately adjacent to arterioles ~50%; Figure 7-10A)

- Less common findings: pseudo cherry ret spot (~26%), macular edema (~22%), and optic disc swelling (~16%)

- Follow-up exam may demonstrate resolution of acute findings, optic disc atrophy, and RPE mottling

Testing

- FA: may show areas of blocked choroidal fluorescence (secondary to the retinal whitening or hemorrhage), non-perfusion (~70%), retinal ischemia (~70%), and slow filling of vessels (~45%); less common findings include early hypofluorescence (~20%), late leakage from ischemic areas (~20%), peripapillary staining (~16%; Figures 7-10B and 7-10C)
- Fundus autofluorescence: hypoautofluorescence in areas of retinal whitening and hyperautofluorescence of retinal vessels
- OCT: hyperreflectivity of inner retinal layers; other findings include macular edema and ellipsoid zone disruption (Figure 7-10D)
- OCT angiography: absent flow in both superficial and deep capillary plexuses

Differential Diagnosis

Commotio retinae, central or branch retinal artery occlusion, hypertensive retinopathy, diabetic retinopathy, HIV retinopathy

Management

- Identify and treat associated systemic conditions
- Visual acuity improvement without treatment is estimated to be 2.7 Snellen lines at approximately 4.5 months follow-up with 50% of cases improving by more than 2 lines and 23% improving by more than 4 lines
- Potential predictors of visual acuity improvement in the first 2 months after presentation include male gender, macular edema, and etiology (trauma and pancreatitis are associated with greater improvement than other etiologies)

8

Drug-Related Retinopathies

CRYSTALLINE RETINOPATHY

Hannah Levin, BS and
Jason Hsu, MD

Crystalline deposits in retina of variable distribution depending on associated condition (Figure 8-1 and Table 8-1)

Signs and Symptoms

Vision loss varies by associated condition and ranges from asymptomatic to mild decrease in visual acuity or color vision to severe vision loss

Exam Findings

Varies based on etiology (see Table 8-1)

Hsu J, Chiang A, eds. *The Pocket Guide to Medical Retina* (pp 219-233).
© 2021 Taylor & Francis Group.

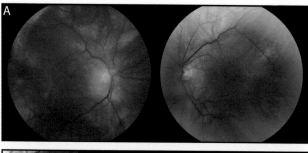

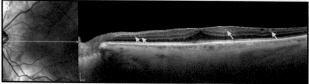

Figure 8-1. Canthaxanthin crystalline retinopathy. (A) Fundus photographs indicate bilateral crystals in a ring surrounding the fovea. (B) OCT shows crystals in the inner retina (arrows). Patient had history of oral canthaxanthin use for tanning.

Testing

- Optical coherence tomography (OCT): depicts depth of crystals within retina and associated retinal pigment epithelial (RPE) atrophy, vitreous hemorrhage, retinal thinning, cystic foveal cavitation, ellipsoid zone (EZ) disruption (Figure 8-1B)
- Fluorescein angiography (FA): determine concurrent findings such as edema, non-perfusion, atrophy, leakage, enlarged foveal avascular zone
- Electroretinogram: reduced amplitudes in select associated conditions (eg, tamoxifen- and cystinosis-related crystals)
- Color vision: may be compromised in select associated conditions

Table 8-1. Crystalline Retinopathies

RETINOPATHY	SIGNS AND SYMPTOMS	EXAM FINDINGS	TESTING	MANAGEMENT
		DRUG ASSOCIATED		
Tamoxifen	Asymptomatic or decreased visual acuity and color vision. Increased risk with cumulative dose > 100 g.	Yellow-white refractile crystals clustered intraretinally in perifoveal macula	OCT: hyperreflective crystals in nerve fiber layer and inner plexiform layer, sometimes with cystic foveal cavitation; FA: no leakage	Lower dosage or discontinue tamoxifen. Vision and edema improve but crystals may remain.
Canthaxanthin (Figure 8-1)	Asymptomatic	Golden intraretinal crystals in ring around fovea	OCT: hyperreflective crystals in outer plexiform layer favoring nasal macula; FA: normal	Discontinue usage

(continued)

Table 8-1. Crystalline Retinopathies (continued)

RETINOPATHY	SIGNS AND SYMPTOMS	EXAM FINDINGS	TESTING	MANAGEMENT
Methoxyflurane	Exposure to now rarely-used anesthetic. Impaired renal function due to calcium oxalate deposition.	Bright yellow-white crystals within or around vessels at RPE level	FA: window defects at RPE deposits	Prevent use; manage associated renal disease
Nitrofurantoin	Slight, gradual decrease in vision after long-term use for urinary tract infections	Circinate pattern of intraretinal refractile deposits in posterior pole, bilateral		Avoid prolonged use or discontinue drug
Talc	Asymptomatic or decreased visual acuity with history of chronic intravenous drug use	Yellow or white refractile opacities inside perifoveal vessels and microvascular abnormalities	OCT: thinning and hyperreflective dots throughout inner retinal layers; FA: non-perfusion, neovascularization, and enlarged foveal avascular zone	Discontinue drug; panretinal photocoagulation if neovascularization

SYSTEMIC		
Cystinosis	Autosomal recessive lysosomal disease → cystine deposition. Vision impairment and photophobia most severe in nephrotic infantile form; milder in non-nephrotic intermediate and adult forms.	In infantile and some intermediate cases, yellow crystals in posterior pole with associated RPE atrophy and mottling. Corneal crystals possible in all forms.	OCT: hyperreflective foci with subfoveal hyporeflectivity throughout all retinal layers; ERG: reduced amplitudes	Cysteamine drops can prevent corneal crystals and decrease disease progression
Oxalosis/primary hyperoxaluria	Autosomal recessive glyoxylate metabolism error → calcium oxalate crystals. Decreased visual acuity most likely due to optic atrophy.	Bilateral macular yellow crystals, often perifoveally, with circumscribed black ringlets of RPE atrophy or lesions	OCT: hyperreflective crystals throughout all retinal layers, lesions within elevated RPE; FA: ring-shaped hyperfluorescence associated with crystals	Pyridoxine, oral citrate, or renal transplant may decrease deposits, but vision loss may be irreversible

(continued)

Table 8-1. Crystalline Retinopathies (continued)

RETINOPATHY	SIGNS AND SYMPTOMS	EXAM FINDINGS	TESTING	MANAGEMENT
Sjögren-Larsson	Photophobia and moderate bilateral vision loss. Systemic disorder is also characterized by intellectual disability, ichthyosis, and spastic diplegia.	Perifoveal white-yellow dot crystals with mottled macular hypopigmentation	OCT: crystals mostly in inner nuclear and outer plexiform layers; cystic foveal cavitation, EZ disruption, RPE atrophy; FA: window defects, enlarged foveal avascular zone	Fat restriction and medium chain fatty acid supplements
Embolic diseases	Transient or persistent vision loss from obstruction of retinal blood flow	White (calcium) or yellow-orange (cholesterol) crystals in retinal arterioles		Testing for carotid atherosclerosis (cholesterol) or calcific aortic stenosis (calcium)

	PRIMARY OCULAR		
Bietti's crystalline dystrophy	Decreased visual acuity, constricted visual field, nyctalopia. Genetic defect in omega-oxidation of ocular fatty acids.	White-yellow crystals in posterior pole and mid-periphery with corresponding RPE atrophy, possible corneal crystals	OCT: hyperreflective crystals mainly in RPE and Bruch's membrane; EZ disruption, loss of outer retina and RPE; FA: window defects, hypofluorescent lesions; ERG: reduced amplitudes	No treatment; disease progresses to severe visual impairment. Associated choroidal neovascularization and cystoid macular edema can be managed.
Idiopathic macular telangiectasia	Vision loss resulting mostly from neovascularization of retina and/or atrophy	Subtle white or golden parafoveal crystals, central sparing ring, associated with macular pigment loss. Subretinal neovascularization and other macular abnormalities may be present.	OCT: hyperreflective inner retinal spots, cystic cavitations and atrophy in fovea; OCT angiography: dilated and/or altered vessels in the capillary plexus; FA: capillary leakage	Treatment with anti-VEGF if neovascularization

(continued)

Table 8-1. Crystalline Retinopathies (continued)

RETINOPATHY	SIGNS AND SYMPTOMS	EXAM FINDINGS	TESTING	MANAGEMENT
		IDIOPATHIC		
West African crystalline maculopathy	Asymptomatic, present in older patients of West African origin	Yellow-green crystals clustered in fovea	OCT: hyperreflective dots in Henle's layer and innermost retina	None
White dot fovea	Generally asymptomatic	Bilateral ring of yellow-white crystals in fovea	OCT: inner retinal hyperreflective granules	None

Differential Diagnosis

Intraretinal crystals—drug associated: tamoxifen, canthaxanthin, methoxyflurane, nitrofurantoin, talc; systemic: cystinosis, Sjögren-Larsson syndrome, embolic disease; primary ocular: idiopathic, macular telangiectasia, chronic retinal detachment; idiopathic: West African crystalline maculopathy, white dot fovea; iatrogenic: history of retina surgery with Tano scraper

Subretinal crystals—Bietti's crystalline dystrophy, calcified drusen, oxalosis

Management

Prevention, monitoring, and treatment of any associated conditions (see Table 8-1)

CHLOROQUINE/HYDROXYCHLOROQUINE RETINAL TOXICITY

David Xu, MD and
James F. Vander, MD

- Risk increases with dosage, duration of use, lower body weight, concurrent renal disease and retinal disease
- Daily dosage of hydroxychloroquine > 5 mg/kg or chloroquine > 3 mg/kg are associated with increased risk

Signs and Symptoms

Early and moderate disease may be asymptomatic; advanced toxicity associated with bilateral blurry vision, poor night vision, decreased peripheral vision, and color vision deficits

Exam Findings

Usually bilateral and symmetric; early toxicity can have a normal appearing fundus or show granular hypopigmentary parafoveal changes and a blunted foveal light reflex; advanced toxicity leads to Bull's eye maculopathy (parafoveal RPE atrophy)

Testing

- Perimetry: paracentral scotoma
- OCT: mild EZ discontinuity early and parafoveal EZ loss and outer retinal atrophy ("flying saucer sign") later (Figure 8-2A)
- Multifocal electroretinography: paracentral amplitude loss
- Fundus autofluorescence: parafoveal hyperautofluorescence early and hypoautofluorescence late (Figure 8-2B)

Differential Diagnosis

Stargardt disease, age-related macular degeneration, cone or cone-rod dystrophy, Bardet-Biedl syndrome

Management

- Screening: patients should undergo a baseline retinal evaluation with spectral domain-OCT and automated perimetry (central 10 degrees with white test stimulus except East Asian patients who should have 24 degree visual field test since toxicity may arise outside the macula) and receive annual screening after 5 years of therapy
- Discontinue at first signs of toxicity as further progression may occur even after cessation of medication

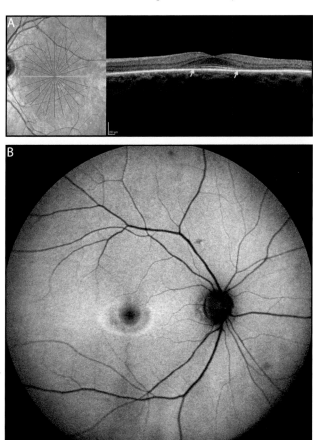

Figure 8-2. Hydroxychloroquine toxicity. (A) OCT demonstrates thinning and attenuation of the parafoveal and macular EZ (outside of arrows). (B) Fundus autofluorescence of a different patient demonstrates parafoveal hyperautofluorescence in a Bull's eye pattern in relatively early toxicity.

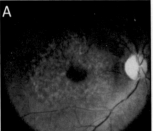

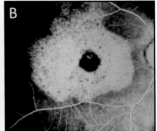

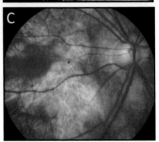

Figure 8-3. (A) Fundus photo with subacute thioridazine toxicity, demonstrating atrophy and stippling of the RPE. (B) FA reveals corresponding well-defined hyperfluorescence consistent with a window defect. (C) Chronic thioridazine toxicity demonstrating a circular pattern of RPE atrophy. (Reprinted with permission from James F. Vander, MD.)

PHENOTHIAZINE-ASSOCIATED RETINOPATHY

Adam T. Gerstenblith, MD

- Pigmentary retinopathy due to drug accumulation in RPE
- Most common with thioridazine doses over 800 mg/day; very rare with chlorpromazine

Signs and Symptoms

Blurred vision early, visual field loss and nyctalopia late

Exam Findings

Early-stage—stippling of RPE in macula; late-stage—diffuse but often patchy RPE atrophy with a characteristic circular pattern which may be confused with choroideremia or Bietti's crystalline dystrophy (Figure 8-3)

Testing

- Fundus autofluoresence: nummular pattern of atrophy of RPE and choriocapillaris with areas of hyper- and hypoautofluoresence
- OCT: defects in outer retinal layers

Differential Diagnosis

Chloroquine-derivative associated retinopathy, congenital rubella, congenital syphilis, Kearns-Sayre syndrome, carrier state of retinitis pigmentosa, choroideremia, and albinism, Leber congenital amaurosis, inherited chorioretinal dystrophies

Management

Cessation of drug may allow for visual function improvement in some cases, though progressive atrophy and visual loss may occur for years afterwards

MEK INHIBITOR RETINOPATHY

Christopher M. Aderman, MD

- Class of chemotherapeutic agents that inhibit mitogen-activated protein kinase/extracellular signal regulation kinase (MAPK/ERK). Trametinib, cobimetinib, and binimetinib are approved by the Food and Drug Administration to treat advanced melanoma with *BRAF* gene mutations.
- Retinopathy is related to acute RPE toxicity leading to hyperpermeability and breakdown of retinal-blood barrier.

Signs and Symptoms

May be asymptomatic; painless blurred vision, distorted vision, altered color perception, photosensitivity, glare, scotoma

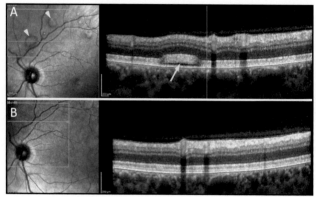

Figure 8-4. (A) Infrared fundus image showing multifocal serous retinal detachments (arrowheads) confirmed on OCT (arrow) in a patient taking a MEK inhibitor. (B) Infrared fundus and OCT image showing resolution within 2 weeks of stopping medication. (Reprinted with permission from Katherine E. Duncan, MD.)

Exam Findings

Multifocal serous retinal detachment, mimicking central serous retinopathy; cystoid macular edema (CME); retinal vein occlusion; typically bilateral, symmetric, and presents acutely within first week after starting drug

Testing

- OCT: multiple neurosensory detachments (Figure 8-4); CME
- FA: delayed arterio-venous transit time in retinal vein occlusion; petaloid leakage from CME

Differential Diagnosis

Central serous retinopathy, hypertensive retinopathy, retinal vein occlusion, diabetic retinopathy, Vogt-Koyanagi-Harada, sympathetic ophthalmia

Management

- If asymptomatic: observe as ocular findings are often self-limited and resolve within days with continued therapy
- If symptomatic: Topical, periocular, or intravitreal steroids for CME. Anti-VEGF agents for macular edema due to retinal vein occlusion. In severe visual impairment, consider dose reduction or temporary discontinuation in consultation with oncologist. After symptoms and OCT findings resolve, patients may be rechallenged at a lower dose.

9

Peripheral Retinal Diseases

RETINAL TEARS

Elisabeth Maureen Sledz, MD and
John D. Pitcher III, MD

- Most common after posterior vitreous detachment (PVD); up to 20% of symptomatic PVD may have tear(s)
- Risk factors: post-trauma, myopia, lattice degeneration, previous cataract surgery, following YAG laser capsulotomy

Categories

- Horseshoe: retinal break caused by vitreous traction; located at sites of strong vitreoretinal adhesion (vitreous base); usually occurs at time of PVD (Figure 9-1A)
- Operculated: round defect with overlying operculum of retinal tissue

Hsu J, Chiang A, eds. *The Pocket Guide to Medical Retina* (pp 235-252).
© 2021 Taylor & Francis Group.

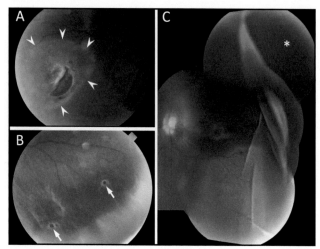

Figure 9-1. (A) Horseshoe tear with cuff of subretinal fluid (arrowheads). (B) Atrophic holes (arrows). (C) Giant retinal tear with a large area of exposed retinal pigment epithelium (*). (Reprinted with permission from William E. Benson, MD.)

- Atrophic hole: caused by chronic thinning of sensory retina rather than traction; associated with myopia and lattice degeneration; may remain stable or cause insidious onset retinal detachment (RD; Figure 9-1B)
- Giant tear: spontaneous or traumatic, >90 degrees or >3 clock hours (Figure 9-1C)

Signs and Symptoms

"Floaters" (spider webs, lines/strings, tiny dots); peripheral "flashes" (photopsias) most prominent at night or in dark room and worsens with eye movement; blurred vision if concomitant vitreous hemorrhage or debris

Exam Findings

- Anterior segment: pigmented cells in anterior vitreous on slit lamp exam (tobacco dust, Shafer's sign); high suspicion for retinal tear if present
- Posterior segment: Weiss ring (circular vitreous condensation); vitreous hemorrhage may be present; retinal tears (most common in superotemporal quadrant, may occur adjacent to lattice degeneration; Figure 9-2)

Testing

Optical coherence tomography (OCT) may show small hyper-reflective dots in vitreous ("falling ash sign") related to pigmented cells or red blood cells

Differential Diagnosis

Vitreous hemorrhage from other etiology, vitritis, pavingstone degeneration, lattice degeneration, meridional fold, retinal tuft

Management

- Emergent laser retinopexy or cryotherapy for acute symptomatic tears to prevent RD
- Asymptomatic operculated and atrophic holes may be observed with education about RD warnings (flashes, floaters, curtain over vision), however treatment may be recommended if history of RD in contralateral eye or strong family history of RD

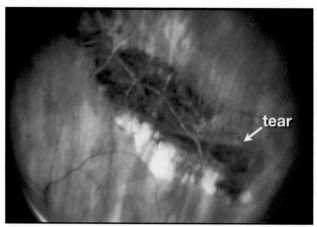

Figure 9-2. Fundus photo shows lattice degeneration with crisscrossing reticular lines, associated with pigmentation from underlying RPE hyperplasia. A retinal tear is noted at the edge of the lattice degeneration (arrow). (Reprinted with permission from William E. Benson, MD.)

LATTICE DEGENERATION

Priya Sharma Vakharia, MD and
Chirag P. Shah, MD, MPH

- Common peripheral retinal finding (~8% to 10% of the population) with increased prevalence in myopic eyes
- Increases risk of retinal tears and detachment, though lifetime risk of RD < 1%

Signs and Symptoms

Typically asymptomatic

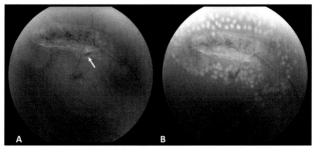

Figure 9-3. (A) Fundus photo of perivascular lattice degeneration associated with a small tear (arrow) at the edge of the lattice degeneration. (B) Appearance of lattice degeneration after successful laser photocoagulation. (Reprinted with permission from William E. Benson, MD.)

Exam Findings

Often located at vitreous base or peripheral retinal vessels and may be focal or diffuse in distribution; variable appearance including crisscrossing fine white reticular lines, snail-track appearance, peripheral perivascular thinning, and condensed areas of vitreoretinal traction overlying retinal thinning; may be associated with pigmentation from retinal pigment epithelial hyperplasia; may be associated with atrophic holes, tears (Figure 9-3A), or RDs

Differential Diagnosis

Cobblestone/pavingstone degeneration, white without pressure, congenital hypertrophy of the retinal pigment epithelium (RPE), RD, retinoschisis, chorioretinal scar, snowflake degeneration, reticular degeneration, normal pigmentation of ora serrata

Management

- Observation in asymptomatic cases: patients should be instructed to return promptly if any symptoms of flashes, floaters, curtain in peripheral vision, or vision changes

- Laser photocoagulation/cryotherapy (Figure 9-3B): consider as prophylaxis in patients with history of RD in fellow eye or if there is documented increase or progression of subretinal fluid secondary to lattice and atrophic round holes

COBBLESTONE DEGENERATION

Paul S. Baker, MD

- Common, benign peripheral RD also known as pavingstone degeneration that is more common with aging
- No associated risk of retinal tears or RD

Signs and Symptoms

Asymptomatic

Exam Findings

Yellow-white round/oval discrete patches of choroidal and retinal atrophy, typically bilateral, often with pigment hyperplasia at edges and large underlying choroidal vessels visible centrally; located in far retinal periphery, between ora serrata and equator, most commonly inferior; usually 1 to several disc diameters in size, and often appear in clusters though may become confluent (Figure 9-4)

Differential Diagnosis

Lattice degeneration, atrophic retinal holes, snail track degeneration, congenital hypertrophy of the retina pigment epithelium (CHRPE)

Management

None

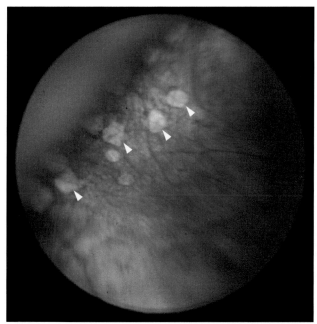

Figure 9-4. Cobblestone degeneration. Typical cluster of yellow-white lesions with well-defined border. Note underlying choroidal vessels within several lesions (arrowheads). (Reprinted with permission from William E. Benson, MD.)

PERIPHERAL RETINOSCHISIS

Roozbeh Akhtari, MD and
David Y. Rhee, MD

- Acquired, cystoid degenerative process occurring in peripheral retina causing splitting of retinal tissue, typically at the outer plexiform layer
- Occurs in ~4% in persons 60 to 80 years old
- Rare complication is posterior progression towards the macula or rhegmatogenous retinal detachment (RRD) via formation of inner and outer retinal holes

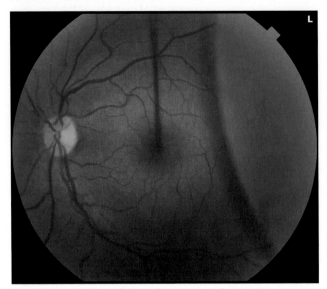

Figure 9-5. Fundus photo of left eye showing temporal retinoschisis.

Signs and Symptoms

Generally asymptomatic, photopsias or blind spot, decreased vision or metamorphopsia if splitting tracks to macula or if an associated RD develops

Exam Findings

Smooth, immobile, dome-shaped elevation of retina without full-thickness holes though small inner layer and/or large outer layer defects may develop; inner retinal layer may demonstrate vascular sheathing or glistening white dots (Figures 9-5, 9-6, and Table 9-1)

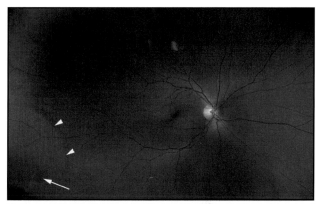

Figure 9-6. Wide-field image of right eye showing inferotemporal peripheral retinoschisis (arrowheads) with outer wall hole (arrow).

Table 9-1. Features of Retinal Detachment Versus Peripheral Retinoschisis

FEATURE	RETINAL DETACHMENT	PERIPHERAL RETINOSCHISIS
LOCATION	Unilateral	Bilateral (~30%), inferotemporal
APPEARANCE	Corrugations (unless chronic) + holes/tears + demarcation line	Smooth, dome-shaped – holes/tears – demarcation line
VISUAL FIELD	Relative scotoma	Absolute scotoma
OCT	Separation of neurosensory layer from RPE	Split within neurosensory layer
SCLERAL DEPRESSION	Separated layers reappose	Separated layers do not reappose
LASER	– blanching	+ blanching

Testing

- OCT: splitting within retinal neurosensory layer (between outer plexiform and inner nuclear layer)
- Perimetry: possible absolute scotoma in region affected

Differential Diagnosis

RRD, juvenile X-linked retinoschisis, central serous chorioretinopathy, exudative (serous) RD

Management

- No treatment for stable, asymptomatic peripheral retinoschisis (applies to vast majority)
- Options for progressive, symptomatic schisis-detachments and associated rhegmatogenous detachments: laser demarcation, pars plana vitrectomy and/or scleral buckle

RHEGMATOGENOUS RETINAL DETACHMENT

Elizabeth Maureen Sledz, MD and
John D. Pitcher III, MD

- Separation of neurosensory retina from RPE
- Etiology: PVD, myopia, lattice degeneration, trauma

Signs and Symptoms

Photopsias, floaters, shadow obscuring peripheral and/or central vision; may be asymptomatic in chronic/slowly progressive cases

Exam Findings

- Anterior segment: mild relative afferent pupillary defect; lower intraocular pressure in affected eye though may be

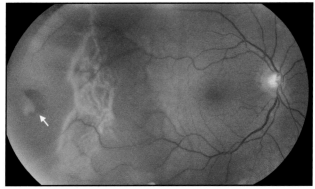

Figure 9-7. Color fundus photo with a temporal macula on RRD. Note the temporal horseshoe tear (arrow) and corrugation in the detached retina.

elevated in chronic RRD (Schwartz-Matsuo syndrome); anterior chamber cells if chronic RRD; pigmented cells in anterior vitreous (tobacco dust, Shafer's sign)

- Posterior segment: elevation of retina from RPE; subretinal fluid does not shift with changes in position; vitreous hemorrhage may be present; in acute RRD: corrugated folds, detached portion of retina appears opaque (Figure 9-7); in chronic RRD: retinal thinning with greater translucency and loss of corrugation, intraretinal cysts, pigmented demarcation line at edge of detachment, underlying RPE atrophy (Figure 9-8)

Lincoff Rules

Helpful for finding retinal tear or hole
- Superotemporal or superonasal RRD: primary break within 1 to 2 clock hours of highest border
- RRDs that cross 12 o'clock or total RRD: break usually within triangle with apex at 12 o'clock ora serrata and sides intersecting equator 1 hour on either side

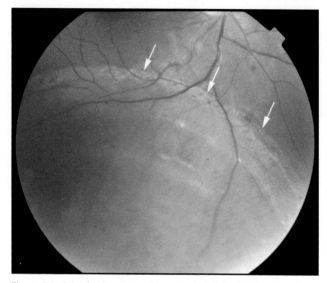

Figure 9-8. Color fundus photo with a chronic inferior RD, demonstrating a pigmented demarcation line (arrows).

- Inferior RD
  - If level of RRD is equal on nasal and temporal side, break is likely at 6 o'clock
    - If bullous, suspect superior break(s) connected by shallow peripheral gutter
  - If level of RRD is higher on one side, break is likely on the higher side

Testing

- B-scan ultrasound: useful when significant media opacities are present; dynamic scan shows mobile appearance in vitreous cavity that remains tethered at ora serrata anteriorly and optic nerve posteriorly depending on extent of RRD; tears may be visualized in periphery; chronic RRD may have an open or closed funnel shape

- OCT: confirm whether fovea is involved in cases of shallow RRD involving the macula

Differential Diagnosis

Retinoschisis, choroidal detachment, serous RD, tractional RD

Management

- Demarcation using laser and/or cryopexy: when macula is not involved and patient relatively asymptomatic
- Pneumatic retinopexy: intravitreal injection of gas or air bubble combined with cryopexy on same day or laser 1 to 2 days later once retina is flat
- Pars plana vitrectomy and/or scleral buckle
- Urgent repair if macula is not yet involved

EXUDATIVE RETINAL DETACHMENT

Samuel K. Steven Houston III, MD

Subretinal fluid accumulation without traction or retinal breaks

Causes

- Vascular: choroidal neovascularization (CNV), hypertensive choroidopathy (malignant hypertension), pre-eclampsia/eclampsia, Coats disease
- Inflammatory: Vogt-Koyanagi-Harada (VKH) syndrome, posterior scleritis
- Neoplastic: choroidal melanoma, choroidal metastasis, choroidal hemangioma

- Uveal effusion syndrome: idiopathic exudative detachment of choroid, ciliary body, retina; associated with scleral thickening that may hamper uveo-scleral fluid egress

Signs and Symptoms

Visual field defect, vitreous floaters in inflammatory causes, absence of photopsias

Exam Findings

Convex configuration of subretinal fluid, absence of corrugations in retina (Figure 9-9A), mobile subretinal fluid that shifts with position, "leopard spots" from chronic subretinal fluid disturbing RPE, choroidal lesions with neoplastic causes (pigmented or hypopigmented mass, vascular lesion), anterior segment inflammation in inflammatory conditions

Testing

- OCT: subretinal fluid, choroidal thickening depending on cause (Figure 9-9B)
- Fluorescein angiography: pattern of hyperfluorescence may highlight cause (VKH, posterior scleritis vs choroidal lesions vs vascular)
- B-scan ultrasound: subretinal fluid; choroidal lesions show choroidal elevation with variable levels of internal reflectivity depending on type of tumor; inflammatory exudative RD may show choroidal thickening in VKH or fluid in posterior episcleral space around optic nerve ("T-sign") in posterior scleritis (Figure 9-9C)

Differential Diagnosis

RRD, tractional RD, retinoschisis, choroidal detachment

Management

Dependent on underlying cause

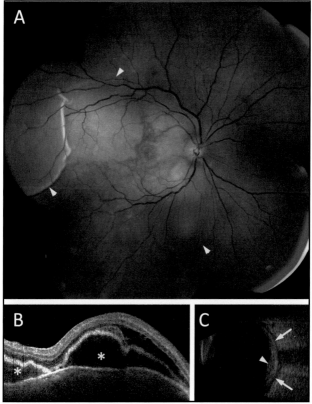

Figure 9-9. (A) Color fundus photo of posterior scleritis with associated exudative RD (arrowheads). (B) OCT confirms serous RD involving the macula (*). (C) B-scan shows classic "T-sign" with fluid in sub-Tenon's space (arrows) and choroidal thickening (arrowhead). (Reprinted with permission from Paul S. Baker, MD.)

Choroidal Detachment

Sean T. Garrity, MD and
Andre J. Witkin, MD

- Two types: serous (due to choroidal vessel leakage) and hemorrhagic (due to choroidal vessel rupture)
- Serous causes: hypotony following intraocular surgery (eg, glaucoma surgery), extensive panretinal photocoagulation, intra- or post-operative wound leak, certain medications (eg, topiramate), chronic RD, chronic inflammation
- Hemorrhagic causes: acute hemorrhage into a serous choroidal detachment, ocular trauma, during or following ocular surgery, spontaneous due to a bleeding diathesis or from abnormalities of choroid

Signs and Symptoms

Serous: painless, variable degree of vision loss depending on whether detachment extends through macula; hemorrhagic: moderate to severe pain, vision loss, often abrupt onset

Exam Findings

- Anterior segment: intraocular pressure usually low in serous type (can be high if angle closure), typically high in hemorrhagic type (if large detachment), shallow anterior chamber in cases of large or anterior detachments
- Posterior segment: smooth, bullous orange-brown elevation of retina and choroid; single or multiple convex lobes delineated by fixation of the choroid to vortex veins (Figure 9-10); hypotony maculopathy may be present

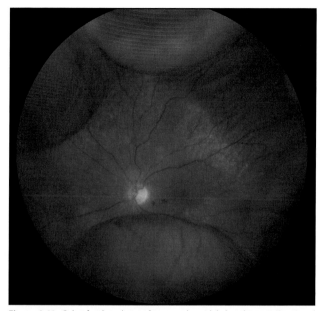

Figure 9-10. Color fundus photo of serous choroidal detachment. (Reprinted with permission from Jay S. Duker, MD.)

Testing

- B-scan ultrasound: dome-shaped contour; larger detachments may consist of multiple domes that "kiss" in the mid-vitreous cavity; hemorrhage appears hyper-echoic while serous fluid is hypo-echoic (Figure 9-11)

Differential Diagnosis

Rhegmatogenous or serous RD, choroidal melanoma or other choroidal tumor, posterior scleritis, angle closure and pupillary block

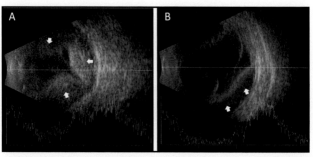

Figure 9-11. (A) B-scan ultrasound with corresponding A-scan (bottom) from a patient with an acute hemorrhagic choroidal detachment, showing the hyper-echoic nature of acute hemorrhage (arrows). (B) Two weeks later, the choroidal detachment has improved, and the hemorrhage occupying the suprachoroidal space has become less hyper-echoic (arrows), signifying liquefaction.

Management

- Typically treat conservatively with topical cycloplegics and corticosteroids
- Surgical intervention if severe anterior chamber shallowing, concurrent RRD or incarceration, retinal apposition ("kissing choroidals"), intractable pain, high intraocular pressure, or persistent decreased visual acuity
  - Hemorrhagic type: generally wait 7 to 14 days to allow blood to liquefy prior to surgical drainage; B-scan ultrasound is helpful in determining the timing, as indicated by hemorrhage that is less hyper-echoic and moving freely on dynamic echography (Figure 9-11)
  - Multiple surgical techniques: external drainage, pars plana vitrectomy, and/or scleral buckling

10

Retinal and Choroidal Tumors

CHOROIDAL NEVUS

Prashant Yadav, MD, FRCS, FACS and
Carol L. Shields, MD

- Occurs in 5% to 7% of Caucasian adults; less common in non-Caucasians
- Rare in children; precursor cells present at birth but do not become apparent until puberty; with aging, becomes slightly larger, with more multifocality, and greater prevalence of drusen
- Small risk for transformation into melanoma

Signs and Symptoms

Asymptomatic; photopsia, floaters, or vision loss if subfoveal (rare)

Hsu J, Chiang A, eds. *The Pocket Guide to Medical Retina* (pp 253-296).
© 2021 Taylor & Francis Group.

Exam Findings

Flat or elevated and pigmented or non-pigmented; overlying drusen and retinal pigment epithelial (RPE) changes common; RPE detachment (10%), choroid neovascularization (CNV) overlying nevus (< 1%), non-pigmented halo (5%)

- Mnemonic for risk of conversion to melanoma—To Find Small Ocular Melanoma Doing Imaging (TFSOM-DIM):

    To (**T**hickness > 2mm)

    Find (subretinal **F**luid, subretinal fluid [SRF])

    Small (**S**ymptoms of vision loss < 20/50)

    Ocular (**O**range pigment)

    Melanoma (**M**elanoma hollow on ultrasonography)

    Doing **IM**aging (DIM) (**DIa**Meter > 5mm)

Testing

- Fundus photography: document tumor features and diameter (Figure 10-1A)
- Ultrasonography: monitor thickness and assess internal characteristics (Figure 10-1B)
- Fundus autofluorescence: overlying orange pigment as hyperautofluorescent spots and RPE atrophy as hypoautofluorescence (Figure 10-1C)
- Fluorescein angiography (FA): hypofluorescence of most choroidal nevi, but occasionally with pinpoint foci of RPE hyperfluorescence on tumor surface (Figure 10-1D)
- Enhanced depth imaging-optical coherence tomography (EDI-OCT): subtle SRF, cystoid macular edema (CME) and overlying orange pigment (Figure 10-1E)

Differential Diagnosis

Choroidal melanoma, choroidal hemangioma, choroidal metastasis, choroidal lymphoma, choroidal granuloma, neovascular age-related macular degeneration

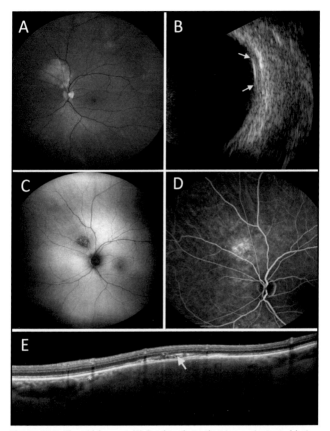

Figure 10-1. Choroidal nevus. (A) Fundus photo showing a pigmented lesion with overlying drusen superior to the optic disc. (B) B-scan ultrasound showing an acoustically dense lesion (between arrows). (C) Autofluorescence showing RPE atrophy as hypoautofluorescence and hyperautofluorescent dots indicating drusen. (D) Fluorescein angiogram showing hyperfluorescence in the AV phase. (E) OCT showing nevus compressing the inner choroidal layer (*) and overlying irregularity of the photoreceptor layer (arrow).

Management

- Typical choroidal nevus without risk factors: observation every 6 months or annually
- Timing of follow-up can be adjusted by number of risk factors present: choroidal nevus with orange pigment, SRF/CME, acoustic hollowness on B-scan ultrasound and those with symptoms are followed more closely
- CNV/SRF treatment options: anti-vascular endothelial growth factor (VEGF) injections, photodynamic therapy (PDT), laser photocoagulation or transpupillary thermotherapy (TTT)

CHOROIDAL MELANOMA

Prashant Yadav, MD, FRCS, FACS and
Carol L. Shields, MD

Most common primary malignancy of eye: 6 cases per million with ~2500 new cases annually in the United States

- Occurs in adult Caucasians (98%); uncommon in non-Caucasians (2%) and children (1%)
- Unilateral (99%) as a rule, bilateral very rare (< 1%). If bilateral, could be related to ocular melanocytosis or BAP-1 cancer predisposition syndrome.
- Predisposing conditions: choroidal nevus, ocular melanocytosis, arc welding

Signs and Symptoms

Vision loss, visual field defect, flashes and floaters, induced hyperopia, metamorphopsia, color vision defect and rarely pain; may also be asymptomatic

Exam Findings

Dome-shaped (75%), mushroom-shaped (19%), or flat (6%) diffuse mass located in choroid; overlying orange pigment, secondary non-rhegmatogenous retinal detachment with shifting fluid, and less commonly subretinal or vitreous hemorrhage; juxtapapillary melanoma can rarely invade optic disc causing disc hyperemia and edema

- Other findings indicative of large tumor/poor prognosis: episcleral sentinel vessels, iris neovascularization, secondary glaucoma, total cataract, choroidal folds, or extraocular extension into orbit

Testing

- Fundus photography: document tumor features and diameter (Figure 10-2A)
- Ultrasonography: measures thickness, diameter and distance from optic nerve as well as presence of exudative retinal detachment and extraocular extension (Figure 10-2B)
  - Classic findings: internal homogeneity with acoustic hollowness, low to medium reflectivity, choroidal excavation and orbital shadowing; mushroom shape, when present, is nearly pathognomonic
- Fundus autofluorescence: hyperautofluorescence of the overlying lipofuscin (orange pigment) within RPE (Figure 10-2C)
- FA: mottled hyperfluorescence in vascular filling phase and diffuse late staining of mass and its overlying SRF; melanomas which break through Bruch's membrane are more likely to show double circulation in which both retinal and choroidal vessels are evident (Figure 10-2D)
- Indocyanine green angiography: intrinsic tumor or dual circulation, mottled hyperfluorescence during the arteriovenous (AV) phase and diffuse late staining of mass and its overlying SRF; hypofluorescence of thin minimal vascular melanomas and hyperfluorescence of larger, thicker tumors

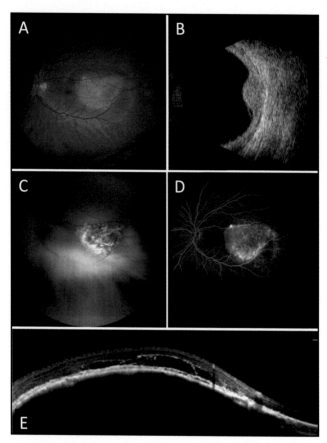

Figure 10-2. Choroidal melanoma. (A) Fundus photo showing a pigmented lesion in the macular area with overlying orange pigment. (B) B-scan ultrasonogram showing a dome-shaped lesion with choroidal excavation and no extraocular extension. (C) Autofluorescence demonstrating lipofuscin (orange pigment) as hyperautofluorescent speckles and layering into a sediment over the tumor. (D) FA showing hyperfluorescence indicating intralesional circulation in the venous phase. (E) OCT showing tumor in the choroid, shallow retinal detachment with debris on the posterior surface (shaggy photoreceptors).

- OCT: Detects SRF, orange pigment and intrinsic features of mass. Also useful in detecting small melanomas with SRF and shaggy photoreceptors (Figure 10-2E).
- Transscleral transillumination: Used commonly for ciliary body tumors. Performed in opposite quadrant to tumor. Helps delineate size and outline of tumor in preparation for plaque application.
- Fine needle aspiration biopsy (FNAB): obtain cytology and cytogenetic results for tumor confirmation and prognostic factors
- Genetic studies from FNAB: alterations in chromosomes 3 and 8 considered high-risk for metastasis

Differential Diagnosis

Choroidal metastasis, choroidal lymphoma, metastatic cutaneous melanoma; choroidal hemangioma, choroidal nevus, posterior scleritis, congenital hypertrophy of the retinal pigment epithelium, retinal artery microaneurysm, choroidal granuloma, prominent vortex vein ampulla

Management

- TTT: used for small pigmented melanomas < 2.5 mm thick in which growth is documented or in combination with plaque radiotherapy in thicker tumors
- PDT: used for small non-pigmented melanomas
- Plaque brachytherapy: used for small, medium, and large melanoma with comparable survival results compared to enucleation
- Charged particle irradiation (proton beam or helium ion): used for small, medium, and large melanoma and has comparable survival rates to plaque brachytherapy
- Local resection: if located in peripheral choroid and ciliary body

- ○ Partial lamellar sclerouvectomy (PLSU): excellent results in experienced hands; supplemental brachytherapy can be then used if tumor is high grade
- Enucleation: preferable for tumors > 18 mm in diameter and 10 mm in thickness
- Orbital exenteration: for tumors showing massive orbital extension
- Combined therapy: plaque treatment followed by TTT

CONGENITAL HYPERTROPHY OF THE RETINAL PIGMENT EPITHELIUM

Prashant Yadav, MD, FRCS, FACS and
Carol L. Shields, MD

Median age at diagnosis is 45 years old; excellent prognosis

Signs and Symptoms

Asymptomatic

Exam Findings

Well-demarcated flat pigmented lesion at level of RPE that can range from a black homogenous lesion to a completely depigmented lesion with majority (88%) pigmented; usually located in mid-periphery and periphery; well-defined depigmented foci (lacunae) in 43%; most solitary lesions have a typical depigmented halo around margin; over 80% enlarge over long-term follow-up

- In rare cases (< 1%) a nodular growth develops, representing adenoma or adenocarcinoma; growth gradually acquires a retinal feeding artery and draining vein leading to yellow intraretinal exudation and exudative retinal detachment

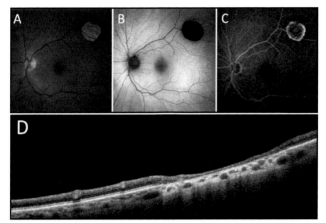

Figure 10-3. Congenital hypertrophy of retinal pigment epithelium. (A) Fundus photo showing lacunae in the lesion. (B) Fundus autofluorescence demonstrating hypoautofluorescent dark area. (C) FA demonstrating a rim of hyperfluorescence in the recirculation phase because of staining. (D) OCT demonstrating thin retina and outer retinal loss.

- In familial adenomatous polyposis, lesions are often multiple and bilateral with irregular depigmented margins forming a fish tail, comma or comet configuration

Testing

- Fundus photography: document tumor features and diameter (Figure 10-3A)
- Fundus autofluorescence: lesion appears dark with no autofluorescence (Figure 10-3B)
- FA: blockage of fluorescence throughout most of sequence; patches of choroidal fluorescence appear through depigmented areas throughout angiography sequence (Figure 10-3C)
- OCT: thickened RPE layer with overlying retinal atrophy (Figure 10-3D)

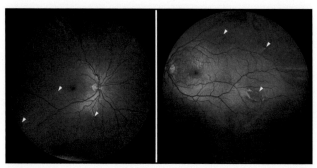

Figure 10-4. Color fundus photos demonstrating multiple bilateral irregularly-shaped congenital hypertrophy of retinal pigment epithelium lesions (arrowheads) as seen in familial adenomatous polyposis.

Differential Diagnosis

Choroidal melanoma, choroidal nevus, multifocal epithelial hypertrophy associated with Gardner's syndrome (Figure 10-4), congenital grouped hypertrophy of the RPE

Management

- Observe as most lesions have excellent prognosis
- Laser photocoagulation and cryotherapy: if a small nodular growth evolves and produces exudation and SRF, laser or cryotherapy can be used to stop progression
- Vitreoretinal surgery: if growth produces surface wrinkling in macular area
- If suspect familial adenomatous polyposis, patients should undergo colonoscopy due to higher risk of colon cancer

Optic Disc Melanocytoma

Prashant Yadav, MD, FRCS, FACS and
Carol L. Shields, MD

Rare unilateral melanocytic nevus occurring most frequently in optic nerve head but may arise anywhere in uvea with mean age at diagnosis of 50 years old

Signs and Symptoms

Most cases asymptomatic; visual loss, optic disc and/or retinal edema

Exam Findings

Dark brown or black lesion which often extends into peripapillary retina and choroid; optic disc edema, retinal edema, localized SRF, retinal exudation, retinal hemorrhage, vitreous seeds and retinal vein obstruction; may undergo spontaneous necrosis with profound visual loss

- Malignant transformation into melanoma occurs in 1% to 2%: progressive growth and visual loss herald malignant transformation

Testing

- Fundus photography: document tumor features and diameter (Figure 10-5A)
- FA: typically shows hypofluorescence throughout the angiogram but may have hyperfluorescence if secondary disc edema or RPE atrophy
- Ultrasonography: thickening of optic nerve and in area of lesion (Figure 10-5B)
- Fundus autofluorescence: hypoautofluorescence of lesion (Figure 10-5C)

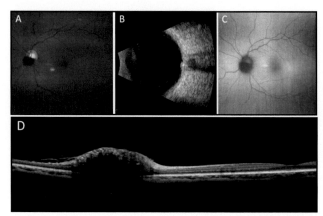

Figure 10-5. Optic disc melanocytoma. (A) Fundus photo with a darkly pigmented lesion over the optic disc. (B) B-scan ultrasound showing an elevated acoustically solid mass at the optic disc. (C) Fundus autofluorescence shows hypoautofluorescence (masking) at the disc. (D) OCT showing an abruptly elevated mass in the optic disc region with complete shadowing posteriorly.

- EDI-OCT: optically dense dome-shaped surface with abrupt shadowing and occasional vitreous opacities (Figure 10-5D)

Differential Diagnosis

Juxtapapillary choroidal melanoma, choroidal nevus, RPE hyperplasia, combined hamartoma of the retina and RPE, adenoma of RPE, metastatic melanoma

Management

- Observation: annual clinical exam and fundus photography
- Enucleation: lesions with documented growth and severe visual loss may be enucleated after confirmation on FNAB

COMBINED HAMARTOMA OF THE RETINA AND RETINAL PIGMENT EPITHELIUM

Prashant Yadav, MD, FRCS, FACS and Carol L. Shields, MD

- Likely congenital, occurring sporadically in normal individuals
- Most often unilateral, but when bilateral, particularly in children, consider neurofibromatosis type 2

Signs and Symptoms

Decreased vision or strabismus in early childhood (most common) through early adulthood

Exam Findings

Ill-defined gray-green retinal mass that demonstrates retinal traction with dragging and/or tortuosity of overlying retinal vessels; classically located on or adjacent to optic disc but can be seen in extrapapillary areas of fundus; of variable size ranging from 1 to 10 mm; peripheral lesions can cause retinal dragging and a dragged disc appearance, and may be associated with peripheral ischemia and secondary peripheral neovascularization

Testing

- Fundus photography: document tumor features and diameter (Figure 10-6A)
- FA: shows markedly abnormal retinal vessels in mass and gradual late staining of lesion
- Ultrasonography: flat lesion (Figure 10-6B)
- Fundus autofluorescence: no autofluorescence (Figure 10-6C)

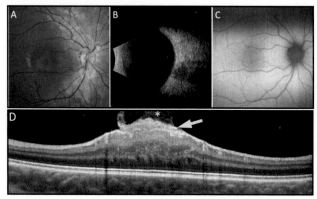

Figure 10-6. Combined hamartoma of the retina and the retinal pigment epithelium. (A) Fundus photo showing a pigmented lesion in the macular area. (B) B-scan ultrasound showing a flat macular lesion. (C) Fundus autofluorescence showing isoautofluorescence. (D) OCT showing folding of the retina, preretinal fibrosis (arrow), and focal vitreous adhesion (*).

- OCT: irregular lesion with vitreoretinal traction in a "saw-tooth" or "folded" pattern that replaces full-thickness retinal tissue (Figure 10-6D)

Differential Diagnosis

Choroidal melanoma, retinoblastoma, choroidal nevus, congenital hypertrophy of the retinal pigment epithelium, melanocytoma, choroidal osteoma, astrocytic hamartoma

Management

- Amblyopia therapy for young children
- Vitrectomy and membrane peeling for cases with vitreous hemorrhage and progressive preretinal gliosis that is not intertwined into the tumor
- Anti-VEGF therapy, PDT, or laser photocoagulation for choroidal neovascularization

RETINAL ASTROCYTIC HAMARTOMA

Prashant Yadav, MD, FRCS, FACS and
Carol L. Shields, MD

- Benign retinal tumor composed of glial cells, predominantly astrocytes
- Congenital in most cases but may become clinically apparent after birth
- Associated with tuberous sclerosis (chromosome 9 and 16), neurofibromatosis type 1 and retinitis pigmentosa; patients with tuberous sclerosis often have 1 or more astrocytomas which may be bilateral

Signs and Symptoms

Asymptomatic and may be detected on screening for tuberous sclerosis; decreased vision if lesion is in macular area

Exam Findings

- Noncalcified variant: gray-yellow sessile lesion in inner aspect of sensory retina; larger lesions have a gray-yellow color and may cause retinal traction
- Calcified variant: glistening yellow spherules of calcification that differ from duller, chalky calcification of retinoblastoma

Testing

- Fundus photography: document tumor features and diameter (Figure 10-7A)
- FA: characteristic network of small blood vessels in venous phase with fairly intense late staining
- Ultrasonography: calcified plaque as seen with an osteoma or retinoblastoma with high internal reflectivity and orbital shadowing (Figure 10-7B)

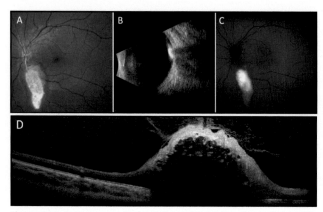

Figure 10-7. Retinal astrocytic hamartoma. (A) Fundus photo of a partially calcified retinal astrocytic hamartoma. (B) B-scan ultrasound demonstrating an acoustically dense and highly-reflective calcified lesion. (C) Fundus autofluorescence displaying hyperautofluorescence of the lesion. (D) OCT showing a "moth eaten" appearance with shadowing corresponding to a foci of calcification.

- Fundus autofluorescence: hyperautofluorescence of lesion (Figure 10-7C)
- OCT: superficial location with highly-reflective features (Figure 10-7D)
- FNAB: confirm diagnosis in atypical cases

Differential Diagnosis

Retinoblastoma, choroidal osteoma, retinal astrocytic hyperplasia, optic nerve drusen

Management

- Observe: majority remain stable though rarely can show progressive growth, exudative retinal detachment and neovascular glaucoma (NVG)

- Laser, cryotherapy or vitreoretinal surgery for proliferative lesions; giant cell variant may cause NVG and ultimately may require enucleation

RETINOBLASTOMA

Prashant Yadav, MD, FRCS, FACS and Carol L. Shields, MD

- Most common intraocular malignancy of childhood accounting for 4% of all childhood cancers; incidence of 1 in 15,000 live births with 250 to 300 new cases a year diagnosed in United States
- Two types: heritable (germline) and non-heritable (somatic). Heritable type has predisposition to non-ocular cancers such as pinealoblastoma which manifest within a year of diagnosis or almost always by 5 years old. Bilateral retinoblastoma with pinealoblastoma is called *trilateral retinoblastoma*. Lifelong risk of secondary cancers, especially osteosarcomas and cutaneous melanomas.
- Presentation within first year of life in bilateral cases and around 2 years old if tumor is unilateral. Careful inquiry about a family history of ocular tumors is critical.
- Survival rates >95% in specialized centers

Signs and Symptoms

Leukocoria (most common), strabismus (second most common); painful red eye: secondary glaucoma with buphthalmos; inflammation: necrotic intraocular retinoblastoma can simulate orbital cellulitis

Exam Findings

- Intraretinal tumor: homogenous, dome-shaped white lesion that becomes irregular often with white flecks of calcification

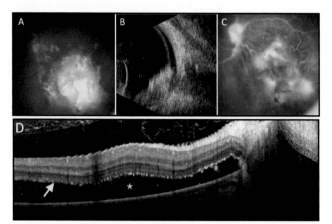

Figure 10-8. Retinoblastoma. (A) Fundus photo showing an endophytic tumor, calcification, hemorrhage, and vitreous seeding. (B) B-scan ultrasound shows an endophytic mass, intrinsic calcification, vitreous involvement, and retinal detachment. (C) FA showing leakage at the disc and hyperfluorescence of the tumor as well as blocking from hemorrhage. (D) OCT shows serous detachment (*) and photoreceptor loss (arrow).

- Endophytic tumor: projects into the vitreous as a white mass that may "seed"
- Exophytic tumor: forms multilobular subretinal white masses and causes overlying retinal detachment
- Diffuse infiltrating tumor: less common and is characterized by flat or minimally elevated tumor growth

Testing

- Fundus photography: document tumor features and diameter (Figure 10-8A)
- Ultrasonography: B-scan shows an acoustically solid mass with highly-reflective foci representing calcification; A-scan shows uniformly high internal reflectivity; useful in differentiating retinoblastoma over Coats disease (Figure 10-8B)

- FA: vascular tumor that fills rapidly with fluorescein and later shows hyperfluorescence; leakage into the vitreous and subretinal space is seen with more advanced tumors (Figure 10-8C)
- OCT: used to estimate fovea and visual potential (Figure 10-8D)
- Fundus autofluorescence: calcification within tumor is hyperautofluorescent; following therapy autofluorescence increases
- Computed tomography (CT)/magnetic resonance imaging (MRI): CT demonstrates intraocular mass with foci of calcification; spiral CT more useful for children as it can be done without general anesthesia and is associated with less radiation; MRI has superior soft tissue contrast resolution more so when used with surface coil and is especially useful in assessing optic nerve involvement and orbital invasion

Differential Diagnosis

Coats disease, persistent hyperplastic primary vitreous, retinopathy of prematurity, toxocariasis, uveitis, vitreoretinal dysplasia, retinocytoma, retinal astrocytoma, endophthalmitis

Management

- Intra-arterial chemotherapy: very effective for unilateral and bilateral retinoblastomas; melphalan +/− topotecan is injected directly into ophthalmic artery via femoral catheter
- Intravenous chemotherapy: vincristine, etoposide and carboplatin for chemoreduction; patients with post-laminar optic nerve invasion or gross (>2 mm) choroidal invasion or a combination of both should be treated with systemic chemotherapy
- Laser photocoagulation: surround small posteriorly located tumors to abolish its blood supply
- TTT: primary treatment of small tumors, but used more commonly during chemoreduction

- Cryotherapy: triple-freeze thaw technique for peripheral lesions
- Intravitreal chemotherapy: used for vitreous seeding; melphalan, topotecan and methotrexate with application of cryotherapy to injection site to prevent seeding
- Plaque radiotherapy: useful when intra-arterial chemotherapy fails to control tumor growth
- Enucleation: mainstay for advanced retinoblastoma with no hope for useful vision

CAPILLARY HEMANGIOMA (HEMANGIOBLASTOMA)

Prashant Yadav, MD, FRCS, FACS and
Carol L. Shields, MD

- May be solitary without systemic disease or component of Von Hippel-Lindau (VHL) syndrome
- Incidence: ~1 in 40,000 live births with estimated 7000 cases in the United States
- Mean age of diagnosis: 18 years old without VHL and 36 years old with VHL

Signs and Symptoms

Asymptomatic and discovered incidentally; macular exudates and retinal detachment may cause visual symptoms

Exam Findings

Reddish-pink tumor in peripheral retina or on optic disc, which may be either exudative or tractional; yellow exudation is often located in macular area, remote from peripheral tumor in both types

- Exudative type: intraretinal and subretinal exudation similar to Coats disease, but distinct red masses with dilated, tortuous, feeding and draining vessels
- Tractional type: similar but also characterized by retinal gliosis, vitreoretinal traction, vitreous hemorrhage and tractional retinal detachment

Testing

- Fundus photography: document tumor features and diameter (Figure 10-9A)
- B-scan ultrasound: demonstrates retinal thickening (Figure 10-9B)
- Fundus autofluorescence: no autofluorescence is seen (Figure 10-9C)
- FA: rapid hyperfluorescence of mass in arterial phase and late hyperfluorescence, often with leakage into vitreous; important to distinguish the feeding artery and the draining vein for treatment (Figure 10-9D)
- OCT: delineates retinal edema and localized detachment (Figure 10-9E)
- CT/MRI: isolate central nervous system tumors and identify systemic associations of VHL
- Genetic testing for VHL

Differential Diagnosis

Retinoblastoma, retinal astrocytoma, vasoproliferative tumor, Coats disease

Management

- Observe asymptomatic juxtapapillary hemangioblastomas without exudation
- Laser photocoagulation: after closing feeder vessels, tumor is treated with low energy long duration burns

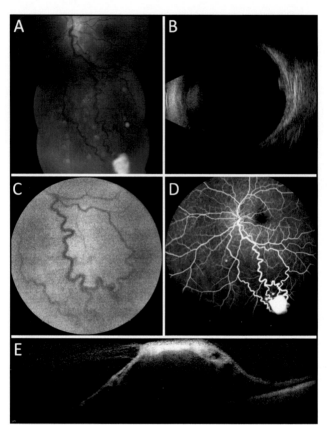

Figure 10-9. Retinal hemangioblastoma. (A) Fundus photo of the peripheral fundus showing a feeder artery and draining vein. (B) B-scan ultrasonogram showing an elevated acoustically solid lesion with no posterior shadowing. (C) Fundus autofluorescence of peripheral fundus shows isoautofluorescence. (D) FA showing intense hyperfluorescence of the mass in the peripheral fundus with dilated feeder and draining vessels without any leakage. (E) OCT of the peripheral hemangioblastoma shows an exophytic optically dense mass with underlying SRF.

- Cryotherapy: used to treat large peripheral lesions with exudative retinal detachment
- PDT and TTT: medium-sized tumors
- Plaque radiotherapy: large tumors
- Vitreoretinal surgery: vitrectomy for endoresection of tumor or ligature of feeding vessel, non-clearing vitreous hemorrhage, epiretinal fibrosis or tractional retinal detachment

RETINAL CAVERNOUS HEMANGIOMA

Prashant Yadav, MD, FRCS, FACS and
Carol L. Shields, MD

- Benign vascular tumor usually diagnosed in children or young adults
- Can occur as an isolated solitary tumor or as a component of an oculoneurocutaneous syndrome that has an autosomal dominant hereditary pattern. Can occur along with choroidal hemangioma and ocular melanocytosis.
- Retinal cavernous hemangiomas may be associated with central nervous system vascular abnormalities, cutaneous vascular malformations; intracranial hemorrhages, small strokes, oculomotor palsies may also occur systemically

Signs and Symptoms

May be asymptomatic; visual loss if vitreous hemorrhage

Exam Findings

Reddish-blue sessile tumor in peripheral retina, less often peripapillary in location; no significant exudation and usually found along course of retinal vein without a dilated feeding artery; white fibroglial tissue near tumor surface; secondary gliosis and traction can lead to foveal ectopia and visual loss; large tumors may cause vitreous hemorrhage and retinal detachment

Testing

- Fundus photography: document tumor features and diameter (Figure 10-10A)
- Ultrasonography: flat acoustically dense lesion with no posterior shadowing (Figure 10-10B)
- Fundus autofluorescence: isoautofluorescence (Figure 10-10C)
- FA: hypofluorescent in early phase; in late venous phase, saccular aneurysms gradually fill upper half of vascular spaces while lower half remains hypofluorescent due to presence of blood; minimal to no leakage of dye (Figure 10-10D)
- OCT: may show SRF and macular edema (Figure 10-10E)
- MRI: investigate systemic vascular anomalies

Differential Diagnosis

Coats disease, retinal microaneurysm, retinal hemorrhage

Management

- Observe as most are relatively stationary
- Vitrectomy for vitreous hemorrhage
- Laser/cryotherapy: helpful for cases with recurrent hemorrhage

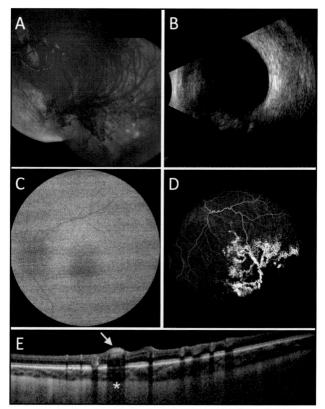

Figure 10-10. Retinal cavernous hemangioma. (A) Fundus photo with overlying vitreous fibrosis. (B) B-scan ultrasound showing a flat acoustically dense lesion with no posterior shadowing. (C) Fundus autofluorescence showing isoautofluorescence. (D) FA with layered hyperfluorescence and grape-like appearance of the aneurysms. (E) OCT revealing hyperreflective areas in inner retinal layers (arrow) causing posterior shadowing (*).

CHOROIDAL HEMANGIOMA

Prashant Yadav, MD, FRCS, FACS and
Carol L. Shields, MD

Two types: circumscribed and diffuse (large and associated with Sturge-Weber syndrome)

Signs and Symptoms

May be asymptomatic; visual loss due to secondary retinal detachment or subfoveal location

Exam Findings

Subtle red-orange mass in posterior choroid that may have overlying hyperplasia and fibrous metaplasia of RPE; secondary serous retinal detachment and retinoschisis can occur over or adjacent to tumor

Testing

- Fundus photography: document tumor features and diameter (Figure 10-11A)
- Ultrasonography: A-scan shows high internal reflectivity; B-scan shows a placoid or ovoid choroidal mass with acoustic solidity; occasionally a highly-reflective plaque over tumor surface due to fibrous or osseous metaplasia of overlying RPE (Figure 10-11B)
- Fundus autofluorescence: associated surface orange pigment and RPE hyperplasia; may show hyperautofluorescence (Figure 10-11C)
- FA: hyperfluorescence of tumor vessels in pre-arterial phase and diffuse late staining of mass (Figure 10-11D)
- Indocyanine green angiography: early filling of lesion and a characteristic washout of hyperfluorescence in later frames

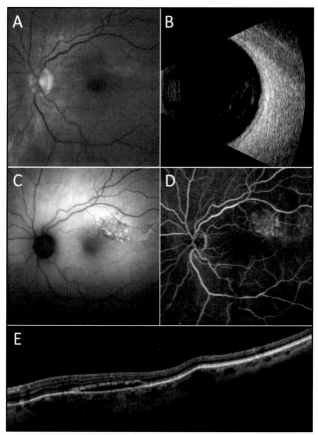

Figure 10-11. Choroidal hemangioma. (A) Fundus photo showing a subtle lesion lying superotemporal to the fovea in the left eye. (B) B-scan ultrasound showing subtle choroidal elevation with acoustic solidity and no choroidal excavation. (C) Fundus autofluorescence depicting overlying lipofuscin hyperautofluorescence. (D) FA in the venous phase showing hyperfluorescence. (E) OCT showing the tumor, SRF, and photoreceptor loss.

- OCT: EDI-OCT reveals a dome-shaped contour with no compression of choriocapillaris; may show subretinal or intraretinal fluid, retinoschisis and retinal atrophy (Figure 10-11E)
- MRI: tumor is hyperintense to vitreous on T1 weighted images and isointense on T2 weighted images

Differential Diagnosis

Choroidal melanoma, choroidal metastasis, choroidal osteoma, central serous chorioretinopathy

Management

- Observation if asymptomatic
- PDT: most promising treatment; standard parameters are used and it may be repeated if SRF recurs or persists
- Radiotherapy: plaque therapy (3000 cGy) or external beam radiation (2000 to 3000 cGy) effective in treating hemangioma associated retinal detachment, especially if PDT fails
- Enucleation: if painful blind eye from NVG and total RD

RETINAL RACEMOSE HEMANGIOMA

Prashant Yadav, MD, FRCS, FACS and
Carol L. Shields, MD

- Benign retinal AV communication that can occur as an isolated solitary lesion or as a component of Wyburn-Mason syndrome
- Wyburn-Mason syndrome: association of AV malformations (AVM) of maxilla, retina, optic nerve, thalamus, hypothalamus, and cerebral cortex

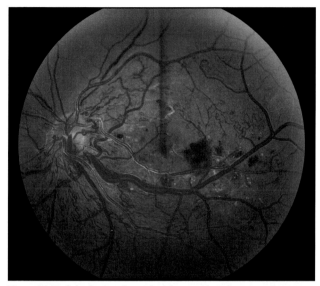

Figure 10-12. Color fundus photo of a left eye with Archer group 2 racemose hemangioma with associated intraretinal hemorrhage and microvascular changes.

Signs and Symptoms

Asymptomatic or cause of visual impairment in an amblyopic eye

Exam Findings

Archer classification for Wyburn-Mason syndrome:

- Group 1: interposition of an arteriolar or abnormal capillary plexus between large communicating vessels; intracranial involvement is uncommon
- Group 2: direct AV communication without the capillary elements; risk of retinal decompensation that can lead to edema, hemorrhage, and vision loss; low-risk for intracranial AVM (Figure 10-12)

- Group 3: more complex AV communications associated with high-risk of severe visual loss; high-risk for intracranial AVM

Testing

- Fundus photography: document tumor features and diameter
- FA: rapid transit and no appreciable leakage of fluorescein
- OCT: irregular retinal surface with optical densities corresponding to the large blood vessels
- MRI: rule out vascular changes in brain and periocular region

Differential Diagnosis

- Retinal capillary hemangioma, familial retinal arteriolar tortuosity, branch retinal vein occlusion, VHL syndrome

Management

- Observe asymptomatic patients
- Rarely vitreous hemorrhage or branch retinal vein occlusion may occur, which can be managed with conventional approaches
- Refer for neurosurgical consultation if associated intracranial AVM

CHOROIDAL OSTEOMA

Prashant Yadav, MD, FRCS, FACS and
Carol L. Shields, MD

- Benign ossifying tumor of unknown etiology seen more commonly in young women
- Unilateral in 79% of cases, bilateral in 21% of cases, mean age at diagnosis is 26 years old

Signs and Symptoms

Gradual visual impairment unless secondary CNV is present

Exam Findings

Orange-yellow, placoid, juxtapapillary or macular lesion with well-defined margins that may show pseudopodia like projections and slowly enlarge; orange-yellow lesions have better prognosis than lesions with black patches indicating RPE proliferation and decalcification; CNV in 30%

Testing

- Fundus photography: document tumor features and diameter (Figure 10-13A)
- Ultrasonography: highly-reflective echo that persists at lower sensitivity along with orbital shadowing due to calcification (Figure 10-13B)
- Fundus autofluorescence: bright hyperautofluorescence in areas of fresh SRF and hypoautofluorescence in areas of decalcification (Figure 10-13C)
- FA: early hyperfluorescence and intense late staining of lesion; vascular tufts may be seen (Figure 10-13D)
- Indocyanine green angiography: may depict intrinsic large tumor vessels and overlying CNV; early hypocyanescence with late staining
- OCT: outer retinal atrophy overlying an irregular choroidal mass and undulating surface topography; preservation of retinal photoreceptors in calcified region and loss of photoreceptors in decalcified region; classic spongy appearance with intralesional vascular channels, bone lamella, Haversian and Volkmann canals (Figure 10-13E)
- CT/MRI: CT demonstrates a choroidal plaque with bone density; MRI is hyperintense on T1 and hypointense on T2

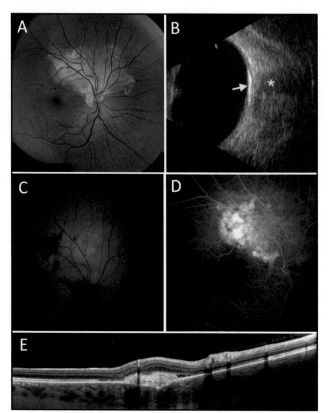

Figure 10-13. Choroidal osteoma. (A) Fundus photo showing a juxtapapillary yellow placoid lesion. (B) B-scan ultrasound showing a placoid lesion in the posterior pole with acoustically dense area (arrow) with posterior shadowing (*). (C) Fundus autofluorescence showing hyperautofluorescence in the calcified part of the lesion and hypoautofluorescence in the decalcified part. (D) FA in the recirculation phase showing hyperfluorescence of the lesion. (E) OCT showing intralesional layers with Haversian channels and markedly thinned outer retinal layer and absent photoreceptors.

Differential Diagnosis

Choroidal metastasis, choroidal melanoma, amelanotic choroidal nevus, posterior scleritis and subretinal fibrosis, sclerochoroidal calcification, intrascleral cartilage associated with organoid nevus syndrome, choroidal granuloma

Management

- Observe asymptomatic lesions
- PDT: used to treat extramacular CNV and induce decalcification of mass if outside fovea
- Anti-VEGF injections if CNV develops
- Laser photocoagulation: barrier laser to limit decalcification from spreading to fovea which may help preserve vision

CHOROIDAL METASTASIS

Prashant Yadav, MD, FRCS, FACS and
Carol L. Shields, MD

- Hematogenous spread: 25% to 30% have no known systemic cancer; 90% involve posterior choroid and 10% arise in iris and ciliary body
- Most common origin: breast cancer in women and lung cancer in men; cutaneous melanoma and bronchial carcinoid tumors also tend to metastasize to uveal tract
- Overall prognosis is poor with Kaplan-Meier 5-year survival at 23%

Signs and Symptoms

Vision changes from macular involvement

Exam Findings

One or more yellow choroidal tumors in 1 or both eyes; frequently arise in macular area with indistinct margins; no inflammation, but can produce serous retinal detachment and overlying pigmentary changes; metastasis from most cancers appear yellowish, except melanoma which is gray-brown and carcinoid, thyroid and renal cell carcinoma which are orange; rarely retinal metastasis can simulate occlusive vasculitis and vitreous seeding; vitreous metastasis is exceedingly rare and most often occurs with cutaneous melanoma; optic disc metastasis can develop from juxtapapillary metastasis

Testing

- Fundus photography: document tumor features and diameter (Figure 10-14A)
- Ultrasonography: identifies lesion underlying an exudative retinal detachment; placoid tumor will show diffuse choroidal thickening; larger dome-shaped lesion shows moderate to high internal reflectivity on A-scan and acoustic solidity on B-scan (Figure 10-14B)
- Fundus autofluorescence: overlying orange pigment within RPE (Figure 10-14C)
- FA: early hyperfluorescence and diffuse late staining; dual circulation (Figure 10-14D)
- Indocyanine green angiography: hypocyanescence throughout the study
- OCT: detects subclinical metastasis and confirms surface topography and invasive features; choriocapillaris thinning and a "lumpy bumpy" contour with small metastases; photoreceptor loss and SRF (Figure 10-14E)
- Systemic investigation: history and physical, mammography, chest radiography and sputum cytology, liver function tests, abdominal and whole-body scans, positron emission tomography (PET) scan, CT scan, fecal occult blood testing (FOBT)

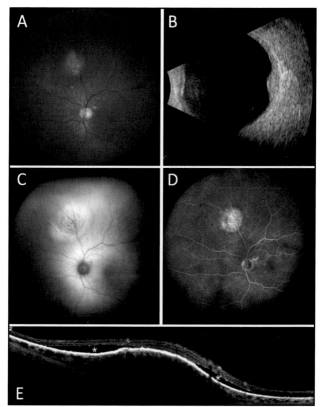

Figure 10-14. Choroidal metastasis. (A) Fundus photo indicating an orange-yellow mass superior to the optic disc. (B) B-scan ultrasound showing choroidal mass with acoustic solidity and no choroidal excavation. (C) Fundus autofluorescence demonstrating overlying hyperautofluorescent lipofuscin. (D) FA in the recirculation phase showing mottled hyperfluorescence of the lesion. (E) OCT depicts choroidal tumor with overlying SRF (*).

and urine analysis; medical oncologist referral if incidental finding with no known primary cancer

Differential Diagnosis

Choroidal amelanotic melanoma, hemangioma, osteoma, granuloma, or amelanotic nevus; posterior scleritis, posterior uveal effusion syndrome, Vogt-Koyanagi-Harada syndrome, central serous retinopathy, subretinal hemorrhage

Management

- Observe small, asymptomatic tumors or those that have responded to prior or present chemotherapy
- PDT for smaller symptomatic tumors in posterior choroid
- Radiation (plaque or external beam) for large symptomatic tumors

CHOROIDAL LYMPHOMA

Prashant Yadav, MD, FRCS, FACS and
Carol L. Shields, MD

- Unilateral process typically affecting men in fifth to seventh decade
- May be primary in uvea or as form of multifocal systemic lymphoma; primary involvement may not have or develop any association with systemic lymphoma
- Most cases represent uveal infiltration by non-Hodgkin B-cell lymphoma

Signs and Symptoms

Progressive painless blurred vision; metamorphopsia if exudative retinal detachment enters fovea; pain if secondary angle closure glaucoma is present; proptosis or diplopia if (+) extraocular extension

Exam Findings

One or more circumscribed yellow-orange choroidal lesions that range from minimally elevated to dome shaped; focal lesions may coalesce to produce diffuse choroidal thickening; some lesions may appear in posterior pole and masquerade as choroidal hemangioma; no inflammation or tumor cells; secondary exudative retinal detachment may be present

Testing

- Fundus photography: document lesions, progression, response to treatment (Figure 10-15A)
- Ultrasonography: diffuse choroidal thickening with low to medium internal reflectivity similar to choroidal melanoma; ovoid echolucent epibulbar mass may be present usually posterior to sclera (Figure 10-15B)
- Fundus autofluorescence: shows isoautofluorescence (Figure 10-15C)
- FA: hypofluorescent in early vascular filling phase with moderate late staining in venous or recirculation phase (Figure 10-15D)
- OCT: "seasick" topography with choroidal thickening and SRF (Figure 10-15E)
- Systemic evaluation: complete blood count, serum protein electrophoresis, CT scan of chest and abdomen
- Biopsy: FNAB of lesion or eye wall in difficult cases; in some cases, there is a conjunctival component that can be biopsied

Differential Diagnosis

Amelanotic melanoma, choroidal metastasis, choroidal hemangioma, birdshot choroidopathy, multifocal choroiditis, sarcoidosis, uveal effusion syndrome

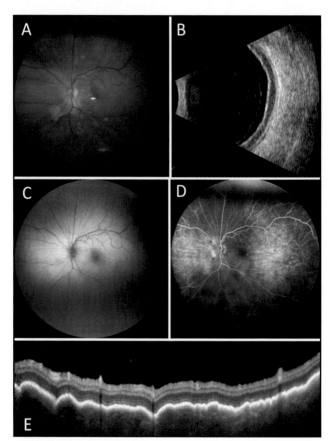

Figure 10-15. Choroidal lymphoma. (A) Fundus photo showing multifocal subretinal pigment epithelial infiltrates. (B) B-scan ultrasound showing choroidal thickening and vitreous involvement. (C) Fundus autofluorescence shows isoautofluorescence. (D) FA showing patchy hyperfluorescence in the recirculation phase. (E) OCT showing a "seasick" topography from thick choroidal infiltration.

Management

- Observe if patient asymptomatic; if known systemic lymphoma and on chemotherapy, monitor closely for regression
- Whole-eye irradiation if patient symptomatic and FNAB confirms diagnosis
- Plaque radiotherapy if lesion is solitary or localized

PRIMARY VITREORETINAL LYMPHOMA

Prashant Yadav, MD, FRCS, FACS and
Carol L. Shields, MD

- Subtype of primary central nervous system lymphoma (PCSNL), a variant of extra-nodal non-Hodgkin lymphoma; ocular findings are initial manifestations of disease in 80%
- Accounts for 65% of intraocular lymphoma and is bilateral in 90% of cases
- Mean age is 60 years old and patients are apparently immunocompetent

Signs and Symptoms

Floaters, blurred vision, red eye, or photophobia

Exam Findings

Anterior segment tumor cells, flare and keratic precipitates; vitreous tumor cells may impede visualization of fundus; multifocal intraretinal infiltrates, retinal thickening with yellow infiltration, round or geographic greasy-yellow mass under RPE, retinal vasculitis, vascular occlusion, exudative retinal detachment, optic atrophy

- Neurological symptoms: headache, nausea, personality changes, motor and sensory deficits, cranial nerve palsies, hemiparesis, ataxia

Testing

- Fundus photography: document tumor features and diameter (Figure 10-16A)
- Ultrasonography: vitreous debris, elevated subretinal lesions, retinal detachment, thickening of optic nerve (Figure 10-16B)
- Fundus autofluorescence: subtle hyperautofluorescence in area of lesion (Figure 10-16C)
- FA: blockage of fluorescence with a granular characteristic due to presence of sub-RPE accumulation of lymphomatous cells ("leopard skin spots"; Figure 10-16D)
- OCT: determine presence of SRF and macular edema (Figure 10-16E)
- FNAB: cytology of vitreous samples or subretinal nodules
- Immunohistochemistry: use of cell surface markers allows identification of B-cells
- Lumbar puncture: may demonstrate malignant cells in a minority of patients

Differential Diagnosis

- Neoplastic (amelanotic melanoma, choroidal lymphoma, metastatic disease); infectious (chronic endophthalmitis, cytomegalovirus retinitis, acute retinal necrosis, toxoplasmosis, syphilis, tuberculosis); noninfectious (acute posterior multifocal placoid pigment epitheliopathy, Behçet's disease, birdshot chorioretinopathy, sarcoidosis)

Management

- Intravitreal methotrexate: requires monthly injections and careful follow-up for tumor control and ocular complications

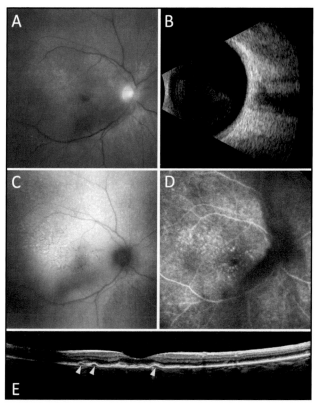

Figure 10-16. Vitreoretinal lymphoma. (A) Fundus photo of right eye showing superotemporal infiltration and hazy media over the lesion indicating vitreous involvement. (B) B-scan ultrasound showing retinal thickening and dense vitreous infiltrate. (C) Fundus autofluorescence showing hyperautofluorescence in the area of the superior temporal arcade. (D) FA showing mottled hyperfluorescence in the area of the lymphoid infiltrate. (E) OCT demonstrating multifocal RPE detachments (arrowheads).

- ○ Intravitreal rituximab has also produced successful results
- Systemic chemotherapy: systemic or intrathecal methotrexate for brain involvement
- Radiotherapy: When confined to eye, external beam radiotherapy (3500 to 4000 cGy) can be given. For concurrent brain involvement, cranial radiation may be used.

RETINAL VASOPROLIFERATIVE TUMOR

Prashant Yadav, MD, FRCS, FACS and
Carol L. Shields, MD

- Also known as vasoproliferative tumor of the ocular fundus (VPTOF)
  - ○ Primary VPTOF: unilateral solitary lesion typically in inferotemporal fundus
  - ○ Secondary VPTOF: occurs in eyes with predisposing conditions including intermediate uveitis, retinitis pigmentosa, toxoplasmosis, toxocariasis, traumatic chorioretinopathy, Coats disease, and familial exudative vitreoretinopathy
- Presents in third to fourth decade with both sexes equally affected

Signs and Symptoms

Asymptomatic to painless vision loss

Exam Findings

Elevated, reddish-pink mass in pre-equatorial region, usually inferotemporal but may occur in all quadrants and posterior fundus; exudation is usually continuous with mass; subretinal and vitreous hemorrhage, RPE proliferation, RPE atrophy, CME, epiretinal membrane

Testing

- Fundus photography: document tumor features and diameter (Figure 10-17A)
- Indocyanine green angiography: hypocyanescence with staining of lesion margin
- Ultrasonography: high internal reflectivity (Figure 10-17B)
- Fundus autofluorescence: no autofluorescence (Figure 10-17C)
- FA: rapid filling of tumor through mildly dilated retinal feeder artery and subsequent fluorescence to lesion; dye usually leaks into subretinal space and overlying vitreous (Figure 10-17D)
- OCT: SRF (Figure 10-17E)

Differential Diagnosis

Retinal hemangioblastoma, amelanotic melanoma, eccentric choroidal neovascularization, choroidal hemangioma, Coats disease

Management

- Observe if asymptomatic as lesions may spontaneously regress
- Cryotherapy if progressive exudation or vitreous hemorrhage
- Laser photocoagulation for smaller lesions without extensive exudation or retinal detachment
- Vitrectomy for non-clearing vitreous hemorrhage along with adjunct laser and cryotherapy
- PDT for smaller lesions
- Plaque radiotherapy reserved for cases that do not respond to other treatments

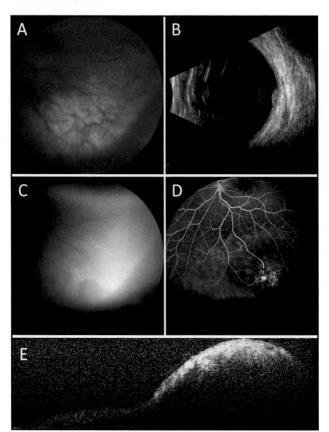

Figure 10-17. Retinal vasoproliferative tumor. (A) Fundus photo showing a peripheral lesion on the left eye. (B) B-scan ultrasound showing an acoustically dense mass with no posterior shadowing. (C) Fundus autofluorescence showing isofluorescence. (D) FA showing hyperfluorescence and leakage in the venous phase. (E) OCT showing an elevated mass with retinal thickening.

Financial Disclosures

Dr. Musa Abdelaziz has no financial or proprietary interest in the materials presented herein.

Dr. Christopher M. Aderman has no financial or proprietary interest in the materials presented herein.

Dr. Roozbeh Akhtari has no financial or proprietary interest in the materials presented herein.

Dr. Tomas S. Aleman has no financial or proprietary interest in the materials presented herein.

Dr. Ferhina S. Ali has no financial or proprietary interest in the materials presented herein.

Dr. Paul S. Baker has no financial or proprietary interest in the materials presented herein.

Dr. Alok S. Bansal has no financial or proprietary interest in the materials presented herein.

Dr. Cagri G. Besirli has no financial or proprietary interest in the materials presented herein.

Dr. Durga S. Borkar has no financial or proprietary interest in the materials presented herein.

Dr. Kevin Broderick has no financial or proprietary interest in the materials presented herein.

Dr. Allen Chiang is a consultant for Apellis, Genentech/Roche, and Orbit Biomedical and receives grant support from Apellis, Genentech/Roche, and Regeneron.

Dr. Jordan D. Deaner receives research funding from Heed Ophthalmic Foundation.

Dr. Michael Dollin has no financial or proprietary interest in the materials presented herein.

Dr. James P. Dunn has no financial or proprietary interest in the materials presented herein.

Dr. Sunir J. Garg has not disclosed any relevant financial relationships.

Dr. Sean T. Garrity has no financial or proprietary interest in the materials presented herein.

Dr. Adam T. Gerstenblith is a speaker for Allergan and Regeneron.

Dr. Kalla A. Gervasio has no financial or proprietary interest in the materials presented herein.

Dr. Shilpa Gulati has not disclosed any relevant financial relationships.

Dr. Allen C. Ho has no financial or proprietary interest in the materials presented herein.

Dr. Samuel K. Steven Houston, III has not disclosed any relevant financial relationships.

Dr. Jason Hsu is a consultant for Orbit Biomedical and receives grant support from Genentech/Roche, Santen, and iVericBio.

Dr. Sasha Hubschman has no financial or proprietary interest in the materials presented herein.

Dr. Thomas Jenkins has no financial or proprietary interest in the materials presented herein.

Dr. Sundeep K. Kasi has no financial or proprietary interest in the materials presented herein.

Dr. Ashley Khalili has no financial or proprietary interest in the materials presented herein.

Dr. M. Ali Khan is a consultant for Allergan.

Dr. Michael A. Klufas has not disclosed any relevant financial relationships.

Dr. Raymond Ko has no financial or proprietary interest in the materials presented herein.

Hannah Levin has no financial or proprietary interest in the materials presented herein.

Dr. Nikolas J. S. London has not disclosed any relevant financial relationships.

Dr. Douglas R. Matsunaga has no financial or proprietary interest in the materials presented herein.

Dr. Sonia Mehta has no financial or proprietary interest in the materials presented herein.

Dr. Phoebe L. Mellen has no financial or proprietary interest in the materials presented herein.

Dr. Eugene A. Milder has no financial or proprietary interest in the materials presented herein.

Dr. Anthony Obeid has no financial or proprietary interest in the materials presented herein.

Dr. Carl H. Park has no financial or proprietary interest in the materials presented herein.

Dr. Samir Patel has no financial or proprietary interest in the materials presented herein.

Dr. Travis J. Peck has no financial or proprietary interest in the materials presented herein.

Dr. John D. Pitcher, III has no financial or proprietary interest in the materials presented herein.

Dr. Ehsan Rahimy is a consultant for Regeneron.

Dr. David C. Reed has no financial or proprietary interest in the materials presented herein.

Dr. Carl D. Regillo is a consultant for Adverum, Aldeyra, Allergan, Chengdu, Genentech/Roche, Graybug, Iconic, Kanghong, Kodiak, Lineage, Merck, Notal, Novartis, Opthea, Santen, and Takeda and receives grant support from Adverum, Allergan, Astellis, Chengdu, Genentech/Roche, Iconic, Iveric, Kanghong, Kodiac, Notal, Novartis, Opthea, Regeneron, and RegenXBio.

Dr. David Y. Rhee has not disclosed any relevant financial relationships.

Dr. Chirag P. Shah is a sub-investigator on trials sponsored by Genentech/Roche, Novartis, and Regeneron.

Dr. Carol L. Shields has no financial or proprietary interest in the materials presented herein.

Dr. Meera D. Sivalingam has no financial or proprietary interest in the materials presented herein.

Dr. Elizabeth Maureen Sledz has no financial or proprietary interest in the materials presented herein.

Dr. Rebecca R. Soares was an investigator for a Jazz Pharmaceuticals sponsored trial.

Dr. Mohamed K. Soliman has no financial or proprietary interest in the materials presented herein.

Dr. Jayanth Sridhar is a consultant for Alcon, Alimera, Oxurion, and Regeneron.

Dr. Maxwell S. Stem has not disclosed any relevant financial relationships.

Dr. Philip P. Storey has no financial or proprietary interest in the materials presented herein.

Dr. Daniel Su has no financial or proprietary interest in the materials presented herein.

Dr. Katherine E. Talcott conducts research for Zeiss.

Dr. Matthew Trese has no financial or proprietary interest in the materials presented herein.

Dr. Joshua H. Uhr has no financial or proprietary interest in the materials presented herein.

Dr. Priya Sharma Vakharia has no financial or proprietary interest in the materials presented herein.

Dr. James F. Vander has no financial or proprietary interest in the materials presented herein.

Dr. Michael J. Venincasa has no financial or proprietary interest in the materials presented herein.

Dr. Eric D. Weichel has no financial or proprietary interest in the materials presented herein.

Turner D. Wibbelsman has no financial or proprietary interest in the materials presented herein.

Dr. Andre J. Witkin has no financial or proprietary interest in the materials presented herein.

Dr. Connie M. Wu has no financial or proprietary interest in the materials presented herein.

Dr. Thomas J. Wubben has no financial or proprietary interest in the materials presented herein.

Dr. David Xu has no financial or proprietary interest in the materials presented herein.

Dr. Prashant Yadav has no financial or proprietary interest in the materials presented herein.

Index

Printed in the United States
by Baker & Taylor Publisher Services